GERIATRICS, GERONTOLOGY AND ELDERLY ISSUES

THE PILATES METHOD

THE KEY TO SUCCESSFUL ACTIVE AGING

GERIATRICS, GERONTOLOGY AND ELDERLY ISSUES

Additional books in this series can be found on Nova's website under the Series tab.

Additional e-books in this series can be found on Nova's website under the eBooks tab.

GERIATRICS, GERONTOLOGY AND ELDERLY ISSUES

TITLE THE PILATES METHOD

THE KEY TO SUCCESSFUL ACTIVE AGING

SILVANA JUNGES

nova
science publishers
New York

NOTICE TO THE READER

The Publisher has taken reasonable care in the preparation of this book, but makes no expressed or implied warranty of any kind and assumes no responsibility for any errors or omissions. No liability is assumed for incidental or consequential damages in connection with or arising out of information contained in this book. The Publisher shall not be liable for any special, consequential, or exemplary damages resulting, in whole or in part, from the readers' use of, or reliance upon, this material. Any parts of this book based on government reports are so indicated and copyright is claimed for those parts to the extent applicable to compilations of such works.

Independent verification should be sought for any data, advice or recommendations contained in this book. In addition, no responsibility is assumed by the publisher for any injury and/or damage to persons or property arising from any methods, products, instructions, ideas or otherwise contained in this publication.

This publication is designed to provide accurate and authoritative information with regard to the subject matter covered herein. It is sold with the clear understanding that the Publisher is not engaged in rendering legal or any other professional services. If legal or any other expert assistance is required, the services of a competent person should be sought. FROM A DECLARATION OF PARTICIPANTS JOINTLY ADOPTED BY A COMMITTEE OF THE AMERICAN BAR ASSOCIATION AND A COMMITTEE OF PUBLISHERS.

Additional color graphics may be available in the e-book version of this book.

Library of Congress Cataloging-in-Publication Data

ISBN: 978-1-53612-174-2
Library of Congress Control Number: 2018936871

Published by Nova Science Publishers, Inc. † New York

CONTENTS

PREFACE

The way we are aging today is dramatically different from our grandparents' experience. That image of a man or a woman hunched over, head lowered, and shuffling along with a walking cane no longer represents the elderly nowadays. This representation, however, is still seen on signage for elderly people at malls and supermarkets.

Yes, we are aging, but in quite a different way. Technological advances and the discovery of new medications have heightened the expectations of a long life. Currently, the ongoing discussion is about how one could increase healthy life expectancy, which is too short when compared with life expectancy at birth.

Basic healthcare of the elderly has improved considerably in the past years, and some geriatric and gerontological centers, in several countries, have sought to develop preventive strategies against aging-related conditions, such as chronic and neurodegenerative diseases.

Given the rise in population aging, there is now a growing concern among government entities about economic and social demands, especially in developed and developing countries. This concern has aroused the interest of health professionals in devising working methodologies targeted at the prevention and treatment of numerous diseases that affect the quality of life and well-being of elderly people.

Nonpharmacological treatment is an alternative that has been implemented by many government entities. This sort of preventive treatment allows for public savings and raises people's awareness about the importance of lifestyle changes. The habit of eating functional foods and practicing exercises regularly has been widely encouraged by preventive medicine and preventive geriatrics.

It is common knowledge that moderate and regular physical exercises are considered by several scientific studies as a preventive and clinical treatment modality for the population at large, but they bring important benefits for the elderly.

In general, the elderly have lots of opportunities at hand to adopt an active lifestyle. Many sports training centers offer exclusive lessons for the elderly. However, the movements performed in generalized exercise routines are intended for motivation and relaxation in a collective group environment. This is very good for socialization of the elderly, but they actually need a specific program to help them overcome physical limitations and have a better performance in their daily and recreational activities.

In recent years, the Pilates method has come to the foreground in the scientific literature, being perceived as the safest and most efficient method for the treatment of various diseases and clinical conditions. Chronic pain, for instance, affects both adults and the elderly. Quite often, this pain causes physical limitations, mood swings and, in more advanced stages, it leads to psychiatric disorders such as depression and kinesiophobia.

Pilates exercises are regarded by several health professionals to be important for maintenance and promotion of physical and mental health at all ages. So far, the positive outcomes highlighted in the scientific literature corroborate what has been observed in practice.

In this book, I expatiate on the foundations and principles of the Pilates method and the importance of applying these principles to the exercises created by Pilates. The book also takes you on a brief but delightful journey into Pilates' life story, showing his devotion to dissecting the fundamentals of biomotor and physiological systems of the human body.

Joseph Pilates was a visionary. By drawing analogies, he predicted the consequences of the imbalance between body and mind for the 21st century. He underscored the importance of achieving a balance between body and mind in order to live in perfect health. He provided new perceptions of the human body in a society that barely cared about health. Pilates conducted several experiments, of which, unfortunately, there are no official records.

Pilates' teachings were immortalized in his books, which include some observations on, and illustrations of, his exercises, classified according to difficulty levels. Despite the scarcity of scientific advancements at his time, his empirical work was highly acclaimed and regarded as efficient by the artistic community, since it permitted enhancing the performance of professional dancers and choreographers, in addition to maintaining their health as well as their physical and mental well-being.

I hope this book will encourage Pilates method practitioners, researchers, and instructors to seek new knowledge and discoveries, which sometimes cannot be contemplated in practice. Practice, knowledge, and research are crucial elements that underlie any successful undertakings.

Now, we perceive that active aging improves the quality of life of the elderly, enabling us to picture them in a somewhat different way: people who have gained autonomy to get about, make decisions, and participate actively in society.

PART 1

Chapter 1

THE PILATES METHOD

In the past 10 years, there has been a burgeoning demand in several countries for the practice of Pilates exercises.

Owing to recent sociocultural changes, the Pilates method has gained momentum, being acknowledged as one of the major exercise routines that promote physical and mental well-being. In the United States, the method has ranked among the top 10 fitness exercises, with the largest number of followers, going from 1.9 million in 2000 to 8.6 million in 2010. In Asia, the method has been as popular as are traditional physical activities such as martial arts and yoga [1].

With such growing interest in the practice of this method, the number of Pilates associations and centers has been on the rise in many continents, and the demand for professional qualification in this area has gone up as well.

Joseph Pilates always believed his teachings would appeal to the masses and would be followed all over the world.

A key aspect of this advancement has been the increasing amount of scientific studies published to date. In the past 7 years, the number of publications on the Pilates method, both at the national and international levels, went up 200%.

However, the method used to be acclaimed only by U.S. dancers and artists until the 1930s. It was only around the 1990s that Pilates' teachings were disseminated as exercise practice among healthcare professionals.

The first followers of the Pilates method were dancers who sought it for rehabilitation of work-related injuries. They eventually perceived that not only did Pilates exercises improve their physical health, but also that they made their technical performance a lot better.

In the first generation of promoters of the Pilates method, we have Eve Gentry (1910-1994), Carola Trier (1913-2000), Romana Kryzanowska (1923-2013), Ron Fletcher (1923-2011), Mary Bowen (1929), Kathy Grant (1921-2010), and Lolita San Miguel (1934). Nowadays, only two of them still live and work in the field.

Numerous elements of classical and modern dance contributed to the Pilates method. These elements ended up influencing modern dance techniques, including those developed by Martha Grahn and Hanya Holm [2].

Despite the increase in the number of scientific publications on Pilates, these figures are rather low.

The empirical research conducted by Pilates was based on a well-devised methodology that was appropriate for the public he investigated. His lessons were planned based on his students' needs and he often utilized some resources to adapt the exercises. The incorporation of the concept and principles of the method enriched his work and the outcomes were often satisfactory. For years on end, Joseph Pilates showed intense and single-minded devotion to researching and developing a method with its own philosophy and based on his studies.

After his death, and after the passing of his wife Clara some time later, there was a dispute over the trademark registration rights. Only on October 20, 2000, following the decision of Hon. Miriam Goldman Cedarbaum, did the federal district court for the Southern District of New York nullify the trademarks, passing the Pilates method into the public domain, for it constituted a working method [3]. Ever since, there has been a remarkable quest for training courses for Pilates instructors.

The Pilates method has become an important tool for the development of physical conditioning and for the treatment of acute and chronic pain, and as corroborated by other studies, the method also brings several benefits to the treatment of neurological, psychiatric, and cardiovascular diseases.

Currently, the Pilates method has been employed in clinical and inpatient rehabilitation. The method can be used in postoperative patients and in patients with chronic conditions, for instance, in those with chronic kidney disease [4].

The exercises are adapted based on each patient's clinical and physical needs, taking into account their individual characteristics. The exercise routines for inpatients have proven to be as efficient as conventional treatments, such as those targeted at patients with post-prostatectomy incontinence or with chronic urinary incontinence [5]. These patients, in addition to feeling the pleasure and well-being provided by the exercises, have a quicker recovery and improve their functional capacity. As a result, their hospital stay is shorter [5].

Today, it is known that, besides the exercise practice and technical knowledge concerning such practice, a method based on scientific evidence is available to health professionals such as physical educators and physical therapists, providing them with the confidence and assurance that they can do a good job.

Given the few scientific publications on the Pilates method – a ballpark figure of 250 articles in national and international journals, more studies with different populations, especially with elderly individuals, are needed to prove the efficiency of the exercises developed by Joseph Pilates.

Chapter 2

WHO WAS JOSEPH PILATES?

Joseph Humbertus Pilates was born on December 9, 1880, in a small town called Möchengladbach, close to Düsseldorf, Germany. His father, Friedrich Pilates, of Greek origin, had been a diligent gymnast with many awards. His mother Haln, of German origin, devoted herself to natural medicine and worked with natural products like herbs and medicinal plants. She believed this treatment was efficient, as it urged the body to heal itself without the use of artificial drugs.

Following in his parents' footsteps, Pilates knew extremely well the influences he had come under. His father's athletic lifestyle and his mother's natural food philosophy and alternative treatments had a profound impact on his professional qualification and lifestyle [2].

As a child, Pilates was too short for his age. He suffered from asthma, rickets, and rheumatic fever. He used to be continuously picked on by older children because of his physique. In his teenage years, he was determined to overcome his physical limitations. Self-taught, young Joseph delved into his studies of human anatomy. He practiced exercises using dumbbells – very rudimentary at that time, as they were made of concrete.

With time, his endeavor paid off. He soon achieved an "anatomical ideal." At the age of 14 years, Pilates posed as a model for anatomy charts. He also took up different sports, including water-skiing, diving, and boxing. In addition, Pilates developed an interest in Zen meditation and in Greco-Roman wrestling workouts.

As years went by, Pilates became known and looked up to for his physique. He was invited to work as an entertainer at a circus. There, Pilates staged the act "living Greek statue," in which he played the role of a man from ancient Greece who was balanced equally in body, mind, and spirit.

Back then, there was no preoccupation with the cult of the body, and Pilates used to be an exception in that society. And that remained so up until the mid-18th century, when the Industrial Revolution gave rise to the sedentary lifestyle. As a result, there was a rise in the incidence of communicable diseases and of childhood mortality, culminating in the decrease of the population's general health status.

In the second half of the 18th century, between 1860 and 1900, countries such as Germany, France, Russia, and Italy also entered into the industrialization era. Steelmaking, electricity, petroleum-derived fuels, the invention of the combustion engine and of the steam locomotive, and the development of chemicals were the major innovations observed in the period. With progress in full swing, aside from other factors, people began to give more and more attention to work, changing their lifestyles. They would now spend most of their time seated. Leisure time became less available and attention to the body was scant – very much like the way we live nowadays, with most of our time spent in front of a computer or in the traffic, rather than actively moving.

Only in the early 20th century, when Pilates reached adulthood, did physical exercises begin to be slowly introduced into social life, through the creation of modern gymnastics – hinged upon the type of gymnastics practiced in Ancient Greece. Its development occurred around 1909, inspired by German pedagogue and activist Friedrich Ludwing Jahn (1778-1852) [2]. He improved gymnastics and turned it into a sports modality. Later on, Jahn utilized equipment as resources (like balls, batons, and ropes) to ameliorate movements. His initial goal was to devise exercises that could help develop strength, dexterity, and endurance, primarily for men.

In the same time period, Swedish physical therapist Per Henrik Ling (1776-1838) developed a new way of doing gymnastics, which highlighted rhythm and flow. At first, his technique was dubbed calisthenics and, later, it eventually became known as physical education. Unlike Jahn, Ling created these exercises primarily for women. Hinged upon an educational approach, the exercises promoted strength, cardiorespiratory resistance, and flexibility. The objective of the exercises was to gain better control over movements and to strengthen abdominal muscles.

From then on, Pilates sought to create exercises targeted at physical fitness, using these teachings along with his intuitive knowledge of the nature of the human body as well as the teachings of eastern philosophy.

In 1914, when World War I broke out, Pilates was 34 years old and worked as boxing and self-defense instructor in England. Because of his German descent, he ended up living as a refugee in a concentration camp in the Isle of Man, UK, throughout the war period.

Faced with the dismal scenario unfolded by the war, Pilates had the opportunity to conduct experiments and apply his knowledge, helping bedridden injured soldiers. He started his tests using mattress springs and strings for the rehabilitation of the patients. As soon as he began experimenting, he perceived that those soldiers who did exercises recovered their muscle tone more quickly than those who were sedentary. Those individuals who exercised also showed larger resistance against influenza and bacterial infections – which accounted for a sizable amount of deaths at the time – when compared with those soldiers who did not do any exercises. It was when Pilates used these makeshift “apparatuses” that he invented the ever popular Universal Reformer and, sometime later, the Cadillac.

After the war, having gained unrivalled experience and solid outcomes from his experiments, Pilates went back to Germany. In Hamburg, he improved his equipment and his method with the help from his brother Fred, who was working as a joiner at that time.

While in Hamburg, Pilates met Hungarian dancer and choreographer Rudolph Von Laban Varalja (1879-1958), who expressed keen interest in his project. Laban shared his knowledge of dance with Pilates in an attempt to perfect classical dance movements, and also to prevent and rehabilitate injuries that were common among dancers. From then onwards, Pilates began working with dancers in New York (USA).

In 1923, on his trip by ship to the USA, Pilates met his wife-to-be and key contributor to his studies, Clara. A nurse by trade, with large experience and knowledge of the human body, she contributed substantially to enriching Pilates' studies. Clara worked closely with him on the early days of his career, devoting herself entirely to his work as a rehabilitator and Pilates instructor.

In 1926, Pilates set up his studio at 939, 8th Avenue, in New York. At that time, the city was already economically hectic with its awfully busy executives and car-filled streets. That scenario did not go unnoticed by Pilates, who perceived the seclusion of man and limitation of his body, which was losing its function to the comfort provided by technology.

Pilates admitted that people were not prepared at the time to be mindful of their health. The perception that body and mind were connected remained widespread only among those who embraced Eastern practices such as yoga, tai chi, and Qigong. He used to say that people would develop some interest in his method only in the 21st century. Pilates was a visionary, because the method went into public domain only in 2000.

Over time, Pilates perfected his exercises by following Eastern and Western teachings. Pilates then developed his method with the aim of restoring the harmony between body and mind. And that's how "Contrology" (popularly known as Pilates method) originated.

At the beginning of this career, Pilates relied on people who had an important role in his life, like his niece Mary Pilates, Fred's daughter. At the age of 16, Mary took on the role of Pilates instructor under the guidance of her uncle, just like his wife, Clara, at the onset.

The first years of his career were harsh. Support from his family members was not enough during the initial years in America.

The stock market crash of 1929, which led to the Great Depression, devastated the economic system worldwide, sparking off a severe crisis in all business sectors, especially in the USA. Because of that, Pilates could not find so many clients, and the publication of his first book, which he had started to write in 1923, was postponed.

His book, *Your Health*, out only in 1934, dealt with functional training, providing instructions on how to keep one's posture in everyday routine and presenting ideas and philosophies on how to attain good quality of life. It was also in this book that he introduced some mat exercises.

His work alongside dancers played a crucial role in his being widely acclaimed, with a promising career. Pilates worked with both mat exercises and apparatuses, aimed mainly at the rehabilitation of injuries that commonly affected dancers.

Numerous classical and modern dance elements eventually contributed to what would give rise to the Pilates method. However, Pilates wanted much more than to merely improve the classical and modern dance techniques. By looking at movements and investigating the anatomy of the human body, he was perfectly aware of kinetic chains and of biomechanical aspects of the psychomotor organization of the human body. His previous work as a boxing and self-defense instructor, in addition to his knowledge of the techniques and philosophy that underlie martial arts, was also paramount to the development of his working methodology.

Pilates was a natural-born researcher. He used to register everything he discovered through pictures and technical drawings.

In 1940, American Ron Fletcher (1921-2011) met Pilates. He was the first dancer to work with Pilates as a contrology instructor. At the very beginning, Pilates helped him recover from spinal column and knee injuries that constantly forced him off the stage. To understand the importance of the exercise routines established by Pilates, it should be underscored that, for choreographers in important dance companies at that time, being kept off the stage meant the end of an artist's career.

In that same year, Pilates befriended some dance professionals: German ballerina Haya Holm (1894-1991), who became a naturalized U.S. citizen; and George Balanchine (1904-1983), Russian choreographer and owner of the dance company, who also became a naturalized U.S. citizen.

It was Balanchine who introduced American ballerina Romana Kryzanowska (1923-2013) to Pilates. At the age of 17, she suffered an ankle injury, which prevented her from carrying on dancing. After some training with Pilates, she had an amazing recovery and returned to the stage.

In 1944, Romana married Peruvian Pablo Mejiane and went to live with him in Peru. During that time, she started a family and had two children.

In 1945, Pilates published his second book entitled *Return to Life through Contrology*, coauthored by William John Miller (unknown biography). In this book, in addition to his philosophies and principles, he introduces a series of mat exercises. The book was dedicated to his wife, Clara.

Thereafter, Pilates worked with several artists from different branches of art.

He provided dance and theater professionals with physical conditioning in a summer camp located on an old farm that had been abandoned during the war. Pilates applied mat exercises to all artists from all branches of dance and theater. The exercises were usually carried out outdoors with a large group of dancers and artists. The summer camp was in Massachusetts, USA. The place was known as Jacob's Pillow, named after the large pillow-shaped rock seen on the property. [6] This dance retreat was inaugurated in the 1930s by Ted Shawn (1891-1972), modern dance pioneer, who set up the Denishawn Company, which was highly acclaimed at the time. He popularized dance forms rooted in theater and cultural traditions outside the European classical ballet. He was influential in training a host of dance pioneers, including Martha Graham, Charles Weidman, Doris Humphrey, and Jack Cole.

The summer camp was an 8-week program. The students lived in sheds or in wooden huts and did all household chores, and also had to make their own costumes. During the summer camp, they practiced dance nonstop, working with a group of famous dancers like Charles Weidman, Valerie Bettis, Iris Mabry, and Devi Dja.

At that time, Pilates was 67 years old and was in charge of providing those dancers and artists with physical conditioning. As usual, the best ones were selected and hired for Broadway shows staged in the subsequent winter (Live, 1947) [6].

In 2003, the Jacob's Pillow property was declared a National Historic Landmark District by the U.S. federal government as "an exceptional cultural venue that holds value for all Americans." It's the only dance entity in the USA to receive this honor. Jacob's Pillow celebrated its 75th anniversary in 2007 and launched its first donation campaign, Jacob's Retirement Fund.

In 1951, soprano Roberta Peters (1930-2017) went to Pilates' studio and asked him to design a series of exercises that could help her improve her pulmonary resistance, physical strength, and stage performance. Using a manual vacuometer (device that measures maximal inspiratory and expiratory pressure), Pilates regularly assessed these functions by following an exercise routine planned to custom-fit Roberta's tour schedules. Over time, Roberta realized she was achieving her goal and felt physically fit.

In 1954, George Balanchine - New York City Ballet's artistic director – was worried about a young dancer named Jacques D'Amboise, regarded as New York City Ballet's main dancer [7]. Balanchine was concerned with D'Amboise's posture and with the bulk of his muscles. He then suggested that the dancer follow an exercise routine designed by Pilates. At first, he was reluctant to follow the training, as he found all the exercises were extremely easy and he felt he was wasting his time. After some time, he noticed the benefits of the method and became a follower. D'Amboise perceived his movements were more harmonious, he could sit down and cross his legs more easily, and he no longer had backaches. Thanks to Pilates' work, D'Amboise turned out to be the main dancer with the New York City Ballet for 25 years.

In 1958, Romana returned to the USA and started working as a Pilates instructor and also as a classical dance instructor.

Pilates was way ahead of his time. He put many years of dedication into his studies and devoted himself to his students. He undertook several experiments in varied branches of human movement science, but unfortunately there exist no official records thereof.

In 1967, on October 9, Pilates died after fighting for his life during several months at the Lenox Hill Hospital. The building where his studio was located had caught fire. In an attempt to save his equipment, Pilates had inhaled too much smoke, which led to severe pulmonary obstruction.

Pilates had a lot of friends and colleagues who looked up to him and were considered his disciples.

Ron Fletcher, a friend and true follower of his teachings, stood by his deathbed and listened to his last words: “My friend, I will stop fighting and give in to death; I am tired, it is time now to be reunited with my father.”

Clara, his wife, put in a lot of effort in carrying on her husband’s work. To do that, she counted on the dancers who had been working with Pilates, like Ron Fletcher and Romana Kryzanowska.

Following in the footsteps of Pilates, Fletcher was invited, in 1972, to work with movie stars in Hollywood, setting up his studio in Beverly Hills, CA, under the name of *The Ron Fletcher Work.*

Fletcher kept in touch with Clara, with whom he exchanged letters.

Clara passed away in 1977. She had held Ron Fletcher in great affection. In his younger years, Fletcher trained hard with Pilates and, sometimes, when he made a mistake, Pilates would reprimand him. Clara used to come to his aid, putting forward her arguments delicately. Fletcher treated her as if she were his mother.

The legacy bequeathed by Pilates spans more than 80 years. He was able to surmount all the obstacles and pushed ahead with dedication and competence. Even though he lived in a time when scientific studies on the prevention and nonpharmacological treatment of several diseases, such as orthopedic and noncommunicable chronic diseases, were lacking, his work was largely known in the artistic community as efficient for offering a higher level of performance in his professional activities, besides health and well-being.

Chapter 3

PILATES: THE BALANCE BETWEEN BODY AND MIND

In the Pilates method, the balance between body and mind only occurs if one is fully aware of each body movement and breath. This conscious balance is of utmost importance to attain the goals of the method. The most important thing is to be aware of what one is doing.

At present, several scientific studies on exercise practice, mainly with respect to those exercises used in Eastern societies, have shown the importance of such balance for the plasticity of the human nervous system. Regardless of age or sex, our body and our mind can heal themselves, alter behaviors, and express our genes.

It is known that the conscious practice of guided and periodized physical exercises brings a lot of benefits to our physiological systems.

The Pilates method has both pleasure and well-being through physical conditioning as a priority. The idea of working all muscles simultaneously and continuously, with harmonious movements, is the most efficient way to improve muscle and respiratory strength. The method proposes to work directly with the deepest muscles, establishing a strong core, without pain, which is usually felt in conventional exercises. The method also gives heed to the perception of one's body as a whole (mind and spirit), which depends on the balance between the physiological systems of the human body and between the human body and the environment.

Pilates, in his first book, *Your Health*, hinges his work upon the benefits and the definitions of the so-called Contrology. He stressed his opinion about the 20th-century man and about his losses and consequences from the failure to comply with the laws of his own nature. He made some remarks about how man developed incorrect posture throughout his physical growth. And that commenced during childhood and worsened gradually from school and college years to adulthood.

In Pilates' opinion, childhood diseases have to do with the way we raise our children, as we often make mistakes that could hamper their development as a whole.

Among his most important remarks, we have:

- Feeding children when they are not hungry;
- Replacing mother's milk with milk formula;
- Overdressing children when they are not cold;
- Forcing children to go to sleep when they are not sleepy;
- Stretching and bending children's arms and legs when they are not prepared to stretch or bend them;
- Compelling children to stand up when they are not strong enough to support their own weight;
- Forcing children to walk when they are not strong enough to control their physical movements;
- Forcing children to sit down when their hip and spinal column are not strong enough to support their trunk;
- Forbidding older children from climbing trees or fences.

For Pilates, children's natural movements are important for their balanced growth and maturation. He used to say that he had learned about the human body by observing animal behavior. He added that compliance with natural laws contributed towards the view that human beings are an integral part of an interlinked system wherein natural selection laws are abided by for the maintenance and evolution of species. Moreover, man, for having a rational brain, should work for the preservation of all species, in order to maintain his own [8].

During his lifetime, Pilates performed many studies and observed human development. He looked into ancient civilizations, drawing much of his inspiration from them to devise his method, principles, and foundations. Pilates used to say we ought to be submissive and governed by the laws of nature.

Ancient Greeks believed that the soul itself was inextricably linked to physical functions and to the manifestation of the mind. They knew the simultaneous development of one's ability to voluntarily control one's body and mind was a fundamental law of nature. They were also aware that the unequal (abnormal) development of either the body or the mind, or the neglect of both, would cause the very first law of civilization – preservation of life – to be a total failure. Should that goal not be achieved, the body would become, so to speak, an "enemy" of the mind, whereas the mind should be a "friend" of the body and vice versa [8].

Recall that ancient Athenians wisely adopted the Roman motto "*mens sana in corpore sano*" as their own.

Chapter 4

CONTROLOGY

Pilates used to say that, in order to realize our capacities to the fullest extent, we should constantly endeavor to have sturdy and healthy bodies and to develop our minds to the limit of our ability.

According to Pilates, Contrology is not a system of haphazard exercises designed exclusively to bulk up muscles. Quite on the contrary. The method was conceived and tested more than 80 years ago and proposes an appropriate and scientific way to exercise all muscles. In Contrology, excessive errors, which are very common in some exercises targeted at developing certain muscles to the detriment of other ones, do not occur. Such errors would have consequences such as loss of grace and of flexibility, or would cause harm to the heart and lungs. Contrology exercises prepare for the development of a strong body and healthy mind, trained to perform all daily activities with ease and perfection, in addition to supplying energy for activities that require greater physical effort, such as sports, recreation, and emergencies.

In Contrology, all muscles are exercised conscientiously. Note that each muscle can cooperate and aid in the equal development of all other muscles.

As Pilates used to say, "Just as small bricks are employed to build and support large buildings, so will the development of small muscles help develop large muscles. [9]" So, according to Pilates, when all muscles are properly and equally developed, there will be minimum effort and maximum pleasure.

Pilates was cognizant of muscular chains and of the relationship between muscle shortening and changes in posture, and was also aware that one or more muscles would be responsible for posture modifications.

The basic aspects of the Pilates method can be summarized as moving effortlessly and assuming full control of one's movements.

Chapter 5

KEY PRINCIPLES OF THE PILATES METHOD

In the late 1970s and in the early 1980s, the Pilates method began to gain popularity when English teacher and dancer Alan Herdman (1941) took it to London and started using it at the London School of Contemporary Dance.

Despite the fact that the method was taught by Pilates' former students, it was also influenced by Philip Fridman, a best-selling author who also published articles in magazines, and Gail Eisen, a former TV producer.

Fridman and Eisen were Romana Kryzanowska's students. Their analytical and writing skills contemplated the need for a book that dealt in detail with the purpose of the Pilates method.

In 1980, Friedman and Eisen published *The Pilates Method: Physical and Mental Conditioning*. The book clearly described the six fundamental principles of the method, namely:

- Concentration: It is important to focus on the exercise being performed; no body part should be neglected at any time.
- Control: To master control of the body, it is necessary to have concentration. All muscles are stimulated to take part in the movement. It is possible to have control at any time and in all movements.

- Flow: Every movement should be continuous like the flow of sea waves. Not too fast, not so slow, always controlling each movement.
- Precision: It depends on concentration and control, and also on body alignment.
- Breathing: Breathing pattern works pretty much like therapy. The purpose is to slow down one's pace of breathing, to take deep breaths, and to integrate breathing with movement.
- Centering: Core stability is the focal point of Pilates method, that is, it consists in correctly controlling the *powerhouse*, as described by Pilates. The *powerhouse* includes the abdomen, hip, and diaphragm, the latter of which plays an essential role in forced expiration. It is the powerhouse that provides the energy for the balance and harmony of movements.

In the Pilates method, the quality of movement is what matters, rather than meaningless repetition, which takes the focus away from the movement. If the focus is placed on quality, by paying attention to detail, precision, and maintenance of movements, pain or straining is avoided.

Friedman and Eisen describe the "ways to find one's body." Breathing, for instance, is a key element in the execution of movements. It makes us aware of the action being carried out and allows us to increase oxygen consumption in all cells.

It is important that the movements be performed simultaneously. Learning the technique involves an educational approach whereby the instructor develops it in a clear and objective manner, respecting the individual characteristics of each student.

Chapter 6

INDICATIONS OF THE METHOD

Physical conditioning is defined as "the ability to carry out daily tasks with vigor and alertness, without undue fatigue, and with ample energy to enjoy leisure time pursuits and to meet unusual situations and unforeseen emergencies." It is a set of health-related attributes that includes cardiorespiratory endurance, muscular endurance, muscular strength, body build, flexibility, agility, balance, coordination, power, and reaction time [10].

However, to achieve ideal physical conditioning, any type of training must be planned and have a specific target. The objectives of the training should meet the specific needs of each student, improving his/her skills at daily or athletic activities and his/her working capacity so as to optimize his/her physical performance.

The Pilates method has become widely known and acclaimed for the fact that it eliminates or minimizes pain and discomfort in bones, muscles, or joints, and because it is a low-impact activity that works with a wide margin of safety, being recommended for any individual, regardless of age [11]. Accordingly, numerous studies have demonstrated Pilates exercises are safe and beneficial, improving the strength and the performance of skeletal muscle, flexibility, posture, and motor and cognitive skills among elderly people [7].

The Pilates method can be applied to the following groups of individuals:

- People who lead a sedentary lifestyle.
- Elderly, pregnant women, children, adolescents, athletes at large, dancers.
- People with noncommunicable chronic diseases, such as asthma, metabolic syndrome, and cancer.
- People with neurodegenerative diseases, such as Parkinson's disease and amyotrophic lateral sclerosis.
- People who require rehabilitation after suffering injury with either acute or chronic pain.

For satisfactory performance outcomes, training should be conducted for a long time period and involves several physiological, psychological, and sociological variables.

Training in both matwork and equipment Pilates must be carried out after a preliminary assessment. Beginners should follow an individualized exercise regimen. This is necessary in order for the instructor to apply the principles of the method and correct basic movements.

It should be noted, though, that the introduction of the principles along with programmed movements has a lot of benefits throughout the training process. Initial corrections are very important, given that, at this stage, the proprioceptive system is activated and muscle tension occurs quickly. During the training sessions, physiological and psychological functions are modeled to accomplish the proposed tasks. Training is classified into three levels (basic, intermediate, and advanced), following a learning difficulty order.

Besides equipment and matwork exercises, other resources are used nowadays to suit the needs of the target public. Different-sized balls with varying density (arc barrel, theraband, tonic-ball, or the magic circle – originally manufactured by Pilates from the metal loop of a beer keg), are employed. These materials are important for adjustment of body alignment, taking into account the student's posture limitations and helping him/her overcome them. For students in this group, the exercises are graded on a personal basis.

For more advanced groups, and those who are physically fit, such as dancers, the number of students could be limited to four per instructor.

Pilates planned his exercises with 5 to 10 repetitions, alternating their pace. He used to say that more than 10 repetitions would make students lose their focus on the exercises as well as on endurance exercises with a set of springs, which demands greater mastery of their strength.

Chapter 7

EQUIPMENT-BASED PILATES

Pilates exercises performed on equipment allow for angle adjustments to find good body alignment and are carried out in a safe and comfortable fashion. This makes corrections easier and enables increasing the intensity of exercises and spring resistance. Movements vary widely, including those that serve an educational purpose, which help with the learning process.

The exercises are carried out on equipment designed by Joseph Pilates, such as the Reformer, Cadillac, Wall Unit, Chair, and Ladder Barrel which, except for the latter one, have a set of springs with different resistance and lengths.

The Chair, also referred to as *wunda chair* (wunda is a corruption of the German word *Wunder* (wonder), was Pilates' last invention.

For movements in which the spring is stretched, spring deformation is defined as the difference between its final and initial lengths. This is called elastic constant of the spring and depends only on the material of which the spring is made and on its geometry, and not on its resistance or deformation. For better spring performance, special attention should be given to the pivot point used as axis so that the movement will have a higher torque depending on the pivot position. Attention should be given to the fixed lever arm, perpendicular to the movable arm. This spring position results in maximum deformation as the movement reaches its maximum torque [12].

The equipment were also designed to help with mat exercises. In addition to rehabilitating human body from the main muscle weaknesses caused by sedentary lifestyle and by the imbalance of kinetic chains, including lack of mobility between vertebral segments, restricted coxofemoral range of motion, stiffness, shortening of hip flexors, and weakening of spinal column extensors, in addition to excessive tension in the shoulder girdle and difficulty in dissipating tensions. These limitations cause spinal column deformations, predisposing to orthopedic diseases.

Chapter 8

TYPES OF KINETIC CHAINS ON EQUIPMENT

The Pilates method employs both open kinetic chain (OKC) and closed kinetic chain (CKC) exercises. Both play an important role in rehabilitation and in physical conditioning.

An OKC is characterized by freedom of the distal aspect, whereas in a CKC the distal aspect is fixed and withstands considerable external resistance, which hinders or reduces its range of motion. Internal resistance can be eventually overcome and, in this case, the distal aspect will move against this resistance.

CKC exercises are considered to be safe and efficient and they have important advantages over OKC exercises. More often than not, these exercises are used with beginners presenting with muscle weakness and postural instability. In rehabilitation programs, this is the type of exercise most commonly used, especially for the rehabilitation of knee injuries. However, a generalization cannot be made. Each exercise has to be assessed individually based on preliminary analyses in order to identify their risks and benefits.

Chapter 9

MATWORK

Mat exercises are usually applied to groups of six or more students. Most of these exercises developed by Joseph Pilates are tailored to a specific public – for instance, dancers and athletes, who have good physical conditioning and good control of their bodies and who know how to apply the principles of the method correctly. For those individuals who are physically unfit, personal training is recommended, with the application of the principles of the method and basic-level educational exercises. The classification of mat exercises follows the same one used for exercises performed on equipment: basic, intermediate, and advanced. Materials such as balls, the magic circle, arc barrel, etc., are used to help students perform movements correctly.

In his second book *Return to Life through Contrology,* Pilates included 34 mat exercises. Ever since, many of his instructors have created their own version of the exercises with a larger number of movements.

Pilates usually taught the same exercise twice (the exercises were tailored to each student, providing him/her with an exclusive program). The new instructors he trained wound up establishing their own work routine.

The adaptation of mat exercises, just as occurred with the exercises performed on equipment, became more intense as the method spread. The exercises were influenced by different areas, such as dance, physical therapy, and physical education, evidencing the tendency towards individualization of new approaches.

Pilates used to say: “It does not matter what you do, but rather how you do it.” This type of philosophy is quite advantageous to Pilates instructors, who can benefit from new ideas, including techniques used by physical education teachers or by physical therapists, targeted at prevention and rehabilitation of injuries, which are added to the method without mischaracterizing it.

The first Pilates method followers perceived that the exercises improved their physical health and technical performance in dance and physical conditioning.

According to Pilates, each mat exercise works all muscles, from the fingertips to the toe tips, as the method never gives priority to certain muscles, neglecting others [13].

Chapter 10

POSTURE

Most scientific articles published to date show significant findings about the positive changes in posture obtained from Pilates exercises. Irrespective of age or sex, these studies corroborate the benefits of the Pilates method, such as pain relief and well-being.

With time, the primary and secondary curves of the spine go through changes. The primary curve has a C shape that is retained by newborn infants. The secondary curves are those developed with growth and maturity (e.g., cervical and lumbar curves). These regions usually demonstrate larger deformity over the years [14].

In general, children have well-balanced and well-centered secondary spinal curves between the ages of 4 and 5 years [15].

Some changes emerge as children grow up, as a result of the posture acquired from daily habits (sitting, lying down, etc.). There are also idiopathic causes, in which deviation is associated with unknown factors that affect bone and joint formation.

During puberty, greater attention to posture is needed because of the growth spurt and of hormonal and behavioral factors. This will impact body structure in adulthood and in old age.

Motherhood also interferes remarkably with women's posture. Pregnancy and weight gain, and later breastfeeding and positioning (how the mother holds her baby) could lead to visible changes in a woman's spinal column.

Posture is classified into static and dynamic; a distinction between the two is sometimes hard to make. It is usually defined as the relative arrangement of body parts. It is a state of musculoskeletal balance that protects support structures from possible progressive injuries or deformities, regardless of the position (upright, lying, squatting, or bending forward) in which these structures work or relax. Musculoskeletal components help maintain the posture, preserving the anatomical structure, the base of support, body mass, and the center of gravity.

Chapter 11

SYSTEM OF MUSCLE CHAINS

The human body functions through a combination of movements. The harmony of such combinations relies upon many aspects associated with posture, such as morphological, physiological, and psychological factors. Postural changes originate from the imbalance in the system of muscle chains.

The life of modern man (with the constant use of cell phones, computers, and, TV sets, etc.) "blocks" our body, causing the spine to bend forward, the shoulders to rotate, and tension to put pressure on the muscles. Moreover, the way the head is tilted forward is also a cause for concern, as shoulder and neck muscles, superior trapezius, levator scapulae, anterior deltoid, chest muscles, and superficial neck muscles (mainly the sternocleidomastoid), are all contracted and overloaded. [16] As tension on these muscles increases, the middle back muscles, especially the inferior trapezius, serratus anterior, rhomboid, and extensors are excessively extended and stretched, whereas the deep neck flexors and suboccipital muscles are weak, and the scapulae protrude and assume a wing-like appearance.

Lower limbs are also affected by poor posture. These limbs provide support and mobility to the body. To fulfill these roles, it is necessary that a good muscular balance of the lower limb be established and sustained. In postural analyses, positioning of the feet and legs (especially of the knees) often reveals shortening and weakening of the lower limbs, and of hip muscles as well.

It should be underscored that hip muscles are closely linked to the spinal column as a whole and that we need the movement potential of the hips as much as we need it for the spinal column. These muscles have to be able to perform functions such as flexion, extension, abduction, adduction, and external and internal rotation. When hips move in this fashion, the joints are lubricated and the correct alignment is obtained, thus preventing daily wear and aiding in hip health and mobility. Recall that the pelvis is connected to the spine. It supports itself upon the hip joints and can tilt from one side to the other, pulling the lumbar spine, which contracts the tissues along the spine. When one learns how to find the neutral position of the pelvis, achieving stability in this region, one learns how to maintain the whole body in balance.

In the Pilates method, for stabilization of this region, one has to contract the posterior part of the lower region of the body, which means slightly rotating the legs, beginning with the hip joint. This slight movement releases the quadriceps and activates the important areas of the hips, glutes, and inner thigh [13]. Pilates exercises are intended to stretch and strengthen the musculature, focusing on the alignments of this region and of superior and posterior chains (for instance, shoulders and scapulae).

Chapter 12

CAUSES OF POSTURAL DEVIATIONS

By and large, postural deviations occur when the agonist muscle is weak and stretched, and antagonist muscles are strong and shortened. Weak muscles allow for deformity while strong muscles produce deformity. Moderately stiff muscles are generally stronger than normal (but not functionally); however, when stiffness is high, strength decreases.

The stretching of stiff muscles results from the improvement in the strength of the weak antagonist muscle, probably mediated by Sherrington's law of reciprocal innervation. This law explains that when a muscle contracts, the antagonist muscle relaxes. This occurs with shortened muscles of the back, flaccid abdominal muscles, shortened hip muscles, and flaccid gluteus muscles [17].

Lumbago (chronic low back pain) is one of the most frequent problems in modern society, accounting for a big share of the public health expenditures in many countries. Epidemiological data demonstrate that lumbago is the most frequent cause of occupational incapacity in the USA among individuals aged less than 45 years.

The failure to establish a definitive diagnosis contributes to several treatment modalities with evidence of success. Regardless of the therapeutic approach, there are several literature references on the necessity of postural correction.

Occasionally, immediate treatment includes alignment correction. However, long-term correction and the prevention of future problems are the most important aspects.

It should be underscored that lumbar region mechanics is intrinsically related to overall posture, especially of the pelvis and of the lower limbs. Stability and alignment of the region result in correction of the pelvis with the diaphragm. The diaphragm facilitates the action of the transverse abdominal, oblique, and multifidus muscles, which are stabilizers of the spine and have a protective activity, allowing for free movement. Recent studies show that specific exercises for reinforcement of multifidi and transverse abdominis help reduce low back pain and stabilize the spinal column.

Note that low back muscles and hip flexors work conjointly to tilt the pelvis anteriorly. That is why the stretching of hip flexors, mainly of the iliopsoas, is important. When the iliopsoas has some asymmetry, it often causes lordosis and lumbar scoliosis.

Chapter 13

TYPES OF POSTURE

Posture is classified into either functional or structural. Functional posture is that which manages to correct spinal deviation when specific exercises are applied. Conversely, in the case of structural (idiopathic) posture, exercises can improve the alignment of structures, but they do not correct the deviation.

In general, when secondary curves, especially those of the low back, show postural deviation, the whole spine becomes unstable.

Two types of posture cause posterior pelvic tilt, extension of the hip joint, and weakness of the iliopsoas muscle. Flatback posture is when the spine becomes straight. The sway-back or relaxed posture is that with anterior pelvic tilt.

A long kyphosis extends to the upper section of the low back and the lower section of the lumbar region is corrected. The posterolateral fibers of the external oblique muscle are stretched. In the sitting position, the area of contact with the ischii determines the level of shortening and weakening of the stabilizer muscles in the region. In general, posterior thigh muscles such as the ischiotibial muscle, and hip muscles such as the piriformis, cause these problems.

When pelvic alignment and centralization are achieved, low back pain is relieved and movements flow easily and are harmonious.

In scoliosis (sideways curve of the spinal column), the curves are C-, S-, or 2S-shaped. These curves are often associated with rotation of one or more vertebrae at the point of the curve. The vertebral body rotates to the convex side and the spinous process to the concave side. The sternum draws close to the convex side. Therefore, the muscles on the concave side are contracted and need to be stretched, whereas the muscles on the convex side are stretched and weak and need reinforcement.

Scoliosis stems from the imbalance of shortened and stretched muscles, but both are weak and nonfunctional. These imbalances cause asymmetric movements and, consequently, poor performance in physical activities. For such cases, unilateral exercises are recommended after a period of adaptation with proprioceptive exercises.

Functional scoliosis is a structural change in tissues, ligaments, tendons, and muscles. This deviation is caused by poor posture usually acquired during puberty and adolescence. This type of deviation can be corrected with exercises if treatment is initiated early on.

Idiopathic (or genetic) scoliosis produces changes in the structure of ligaments, bones, and muscles. Adequate exercises can improve alignment of the structures, but they may not correct the deviation completely. A simplified clinical examination of the spinal column can be carried out by health professionals for initial screening of idiopathic scoliosis, consisting mainly of the Adams' forward bend test, Thales angle, and the inferior scapular angle.

Kyphosis, just as other spinal deformities, can be classified as congenital, associated with systemic diseases, senile, and juvenile. The curve is considered to be physiological when it is mobile and compressed at 20 to 40 degrees. If it exceeds these angles, it is called hyperkyphosis. The level of kyphosis is determined by the Cobb technique. This world-acclaimed technique is based on the angle formed by the straight lines that run from the lines that are tangent to the upper and lower surfaces of the vertebra and that reach further towards the center of the concavity of the curve [17].

Severe hyperkyphosis produces pressure on the lower ribs towards the pelvis, usually causing pain and tension in iliocostal muscles. In many cases, this eventually reduces respiratory capacity and leads to chronic respiratory problems.

Postural analyses reveal that excessive curvature and the forward positioning of the head reduces stature which, according to some studies, ranges from 6 to 11% per decade in those aged over 55 years, and poses risks of fractures, irrespective of bone mineral density [14].

In postmenopausal women with hyperkyphosis greater than 50 degrees, there is remarkable reduction of the subacromial space. Scapular malposition causes deformity in the acromion, thereby reducing this space and shoulder extension as well [14].

In elderly people, shoulder injuries differ from those observed among young individuals who perform the same activities. Kinetics is exactly the same, and so are mechanical stresses on the shoulder, but there are striking differences in shoulder structures that result from aging and posture.

Quite often, sedentary postmenopausal women have modifications in their thoracic curvature and an increase in the degree of kyphosis. This affects cardiopulmonary function, in addition to the whole body structure, including axial and pelvic alignment. As a consequence, there is gait imbalance, reduction in daily abilities, and decline in physical conditioning. Metabolic functions are also compromised, which could eventually increase mortality rates.

Studies have demonstrated that physically active people are at a lower risk for kyphosis than their sedentary counterparts, as spinal extension exercises can reduce spinal deformity or delay deformation [14].

In 2009, I carried out a study on the efficacy of Pilates method in the treatment of adult women with hyperkyphosis. I obtained results with significant and surprising differences between the groups that participated in the study. I treated a group of 41 women (mean age of 60 years) with hyperkyphosis for seven months. The degree of kyphosis decreased by 8 degrees, on average, in the experimental group. However, the case of a volunteer with 14 degrees of kyphosis, assessed before and after the intervention, stood out from the rest. Besides the reduction in the degree of kyphosis, the experimental group also gained height (average of 1 cm).

This change is hypothetically related to the alterations observed in the spinal curves, especially in the thoracic region.

Chapter 14

Posture and Pain

Seeking treatment for alleviation of pain, chiefly back pain, dates back to the Ancient East times. Nevertheless, the major influence upon western civilization came from Hippocrates (460 to 377 BC) and Galeno (131 to 201 AD).

In the early Greek times, the Hippocratic medical school devised ingenious methods for treating common lumbar spine problems. Their methods included procedures for pain relief in lower lumbar vertebral luxations. The techniques were very rudimentary, and included placing patients upside down with their feet tied with ropes and the body strapped to a backrest-like structure. The patients were kept in this position for a given time [17].

Galeno followed the precepts of the Hippocratic medicine, which was built upon a logical science based on experimentation and observation. He developed rehabilitation therapies and exercise regimens, including the treatment for shoulder luxation [17].

Chapter 15

WHAT IS PAIN?

Pain prompts us to avoid situations that could harm our bodies, acting as if it were a "fire alarm." We can refer to this "alarm" as nociceptors. Nociceptors are activated by stimuli that could potentially injure tissues. Most nociceptors respond to mechanical, thermal, and chemical stimuli. They are known as polymodal nociceptors [18].

During daily activities, low levels of nociceptive activity are important as they indicate us when a certain movement or prolonged posture is causing any stress to our body. Even while we are sleeping, nociception can be a determining factor that prompts us to change positions in bed, thereby preventing bedsores or excess tension on the skeleton.

During a strenuous activity, as in a marathon, when tissue oxygen level is lower than oxygen demand, cells use anaerobic metabolism to produce ATP (energy storage), and lactic acid eventually accumulates. Such accumulation leads to an excessive amount of $H+$ ions in the extracellular fluid. These ions activate $H+$-dependent ion channels in nociceptors. This mechanism is what causes the intense pain associated with strenuous exercises [19].

When we increase or eliminate the physiological curvature of our spine, we are predisposed to backache, and there could be some muscle contracture or spasm.

There exist several potential pain triggers in spinal pain syndromes, and most times the anatomic structure does not make any difference. The functional stabilization training fundamentals are proportional to the awareness of movements, knowledge of safe postures, functional strength, and coordination to exert control over spinal diffusion.

In order to understand pain caused by poor posture, it is crucial to know that the cumulative effects of small stresses that occur constantly or are recurrent for a long time period may give rise to the same problems that result from sudden and intense stress. Continuous stress is also known as chronic pain, and its treatment takes longer and relies on changes in neurological patterns. The onset and severity of postural pain vary considerably. In some cases, there are only acute symptoms, usually as a result of unusual stress or injury. In some other cases, the onset is acute and there are chronic painful symptoms. Yet other cases have chronic symptoms that become acute later.

There are striking differences between the treatment of an acute painful condition and that of a chronic condition. A given procedure may be acknowledged and accepted as therapeutic when applied at the right time. If the time is not right, the same procedure could be inefficient or even harmful. Emotional stress can cause acute pain initially followed by muscle spasm. The problem can be just temporary or stress can last longer and develop into a chronic condition.

Chronic neck pain can be caused by poor posture in the dorsal region. One of the main characteristics of this region is its predisposition to stress and to severe injury. The same applies to the lumbar region, which is influenced by the poor posture of the dorsal region and relies on the positioning of the pelvis and of joint, muscular, and neurologic structures.

Regarding the characteristics of muscle fibers, slow twitch fibers (red fibers) are usually monoarticular, smaller, dense, and can withstand a recurrent position for a longer time. That is why they are more prone to shortening, stiffness, and compressive pain. These negative adaptations can compress nerve structures and affect posture.

Current studies have indicated that myofascial release is an alternative option for the treatment of muscle pain, which could possible become chronic. When muscles are weak and cannot bear loads, or when they are strong but show poor elasticity, they can develop knots.

In general, healthy muscles do not have stiff bundles and their fasciae are spared from spasms, stiffness, and tension; therefore, they have no knots and/or pain on palpation [15].

When muscle bundles are stiff and have painful areas, a syndrome known as myofibrosis or fibromyalgia, "trigger point" or "tender point" could develop. The names may vary depending on its severity and on the status of the muscles. The myofascial pain syndrome has fewer painful spots than does fibromyalgia, which is characterized by referred pain (trigger point) or localized pain (tender point), morning stiffness, sleep disorders, anxiety, etc. Its etiology could be related to degenerative diseases, such as rheumatism, stress, etc.

Clinical treatment is indicated according to each case and it is aimed at eliminating the knots and relieving the pain. Once stiffness and active knots are eliminated, it is advisable that the muscles affected by stiffness be slightly stretched.

Note that the key objective of the Pilates method is to allow students to exert control over their own bodies. So, it is important that the process be didactic and based on active participation. Perception of postural habits and knowledge of concepts and anatomical principles, in easy-to-understand language, allow students to take part in the rehabilitation of their injuries and in their body building process.

During events of acute or chronic pain, the use of inappropriate expressions has a remarkable impact on patients. Hence, for application of the exercises, the instructor should prioritize the teaching of the basic principles of the method.

Most studies published to date deal with low back pain. And they all corroborate the positive outcomes obtained with the Pilates method.

On the other hand, there is a paucity of studies that assess exercises performed on equipment; most studies investigate mat exercises (mat Pilates).

For Da Luz et al., (2014), exercises performed on equipment may be more efficient than mat workouts, since they have a medium-term effect on deficient movements and on kinesiophobia.

I believe the spring system used by the equipment, besides comfort and safety, allows for better control and flow of movements. The equipment also employ different-sized benches to provide the alignment that is necessary when performing the exercises. Further investigation is needed, though.

The spinal column is susceptible to changes over time and subject to pain caused by such changes, in addition to other factors associated with aging.

Advanced age and sedentary lifestyle may lead to the disuse syndrome – also called immobility syndrome. This syndrome consists of a constellation of signs and symptoms triggered by the suppression of all joint movements and, consequently, by the inability to keep one's posture. [20]

The Pilates method plays an important role in the prevention of musculoskeletal disorders.

Pilates exercises have gained popularity in the scientific community owing to its safety and efficacy in different populations, including the elderly and unhealthy or debilitated patients.

Chapter 16

BENEFITS FOR PHYSIOLOGICAL SYSTEMS

In old age, physiological functions are reduced and could make individuals more vulnerable to aging-associated diseases. However, with age, the body may acquire strategies to improve physiological functions (e.g., functions of cardiac and immunological systems).

The maintenance of functionality of the musculoskeletal system requires stimuli through physical activities and regular physical exercises throughout life, in addition to nutritional care by a health professional in major stages, such as during growth, reproduction, and aging.

The Pilates method plays a key role in physiological systems. We can say that exercises regulate these systems, preventing aging-associated diseases, especially those affecting the neuromuscular and cardiac systems. Aside from prevention, the method also has significant outcomes related to the treatment of these diseases.

Our body consists of several physiological systems that work together, ensuring homeostasis. Homeostasis is the ability of living systems to self-regulate their internal environment, maintaining the body stable, even in the presence of external aggressive events that could upset this stability. When homeostasis is lost, the ability to adapt to intrinsic and extrinsic aggressive events is compromised, increasing vulnerability to diseases. In what follows, we discuss the major systems affected by the aging process, inactivity, and associated diseases.

Chapter 17

CARDIOVASCULAR SYSTEM

All physiological functions and virtually all cells in the human body depend, to some extent, on the circulatory system, also referred to as cardiovascular system. The cardiovascular system is composed of the heart (cardio) and vascular components (arteries, arterioles, capillaries, venules, and veins), and blood.

It is practically impossible to refer to this system without mentioning cardiorespiratory function and its performance.

The cardiovascular system allows the transport of oxygen and hormones to the cells throughout the body and the elimination of carbon dioxide and of metabolic products.

The heart is the central pump for the system, carrying blood throughout the body. The cardiac muscle, also called myocardium, has different thicknesses within the heart, which vary according to the pressure made against its walls. The left ventricle is considered to be the strongest chamber as, on many occasions, it has to contract to generate enough pressure and pump blood through the body. When we are sitting or standing, the left ventricle has to have a strong enough contraction to overcome the effect of gravity, which tends to make blood accumulate in lower extremities. During physical exercises (whether aerobic or endurance), there is more left ventricle strain, which results in larger thickness of its muscle wall – a process known as hypertrophy. In contrast with the positive changes obtained from physical training, the myocardium can also become hypertrophic because of diseases such as cardiac valvulopathy and high blood pressure [19].

Whether we are at rest or under normal conditions, the cardiovascular system works constantly to meet the demands from tissues. The tissues that are more metabolically active receive the largest blood supply. To have an idea, under normal conditions and at rest, the liver and the kidneys, together, receive approximately half of the circulating blood (27 and 22%, respectively), whereas the musculoskeletal muscle receives around 15%. [19] On the other hand, when we are doing exercises, the cardiovascular system has larger and more urgent demands. During exercise, blood is pumped to areas that need it more. In a race, for example, this distribution increases remarkably. The muscles receive 80% or more blood. This occurs through higher cardiac output, increasing the blood flow to active muscles by up to 25 times [19].

However, it should be noted that this process occurs in intense exercises, usually performed by athletes. In the Pilates method, exercises are moderate and controlled, though, as they are usually practiced by individuals who seek physical conditioning and well-being. According to the most recent recommendations made by the ACSM (American College of Sports Medicine, 2010), in order for adults and elderly to stay healthy, it is necessary that they practice moderate exercises that are gradually progressive and not participate in competitions [21].

The difference with respect to the Pilates method for other types of moderate and endurance exercises lies in the performance of breathing exercises along with the movements. Some basic exercises (for instance, footwork) are very important, as their movements serve as a pumping system, helping the whole circulatory system and cardiac functions, as in the activity of the left ventricle. As muscles contract, they compress the veins and help blood return to the heart. The valves, present within the veins, guarantee the one-directional flow of blood back to the heart.

In the respiratory chain, the diaphragm and the abdominal muscles also play important roles in venous return. To have a better understanding of this pumping system, in anatomic terms, recall that the diaphragm is located in the costal and lumbar regions (L1 to L4), adjacent to the iliopsoas. When we perform forced expiration, these muscles, together with the pelvic floor muscles, "milk" the vena cava and the inferior aorta. This mechanism enhances the efficiency of venous return and strengthens the muscles in the region, preventing urinary disorders and improving spinal column stability. Thus, we can classify the diaphragm (adjacent to the abdominal muscles) as the "second pumping system."

Regardless of the type of physical activity or physical exercise, the activated muscles somehow help with venous return. In Pilates exercises, this group of muscles, known as "powerhouse," is constantly activated, as well as leg muscles, where the gastrocnemius and soleus are recruited at regular frequency.

When we spend a lot of time standing, the cardiovascular system needs help to overcome the force of gravity and make blood return from the lower extremities to the heart. These basic mechanisms are therefore essential as they make the valves and the muscles in the posterior chain work more efficiently.

In his studies, Pilates counted on his life experience and on the observation of the results of his work throughout the years. He believed an adult individual with strong heart and muscles guarded the secret to longevity. He underscored that contrology exercises carried pure and fresh blood to each muscle fiber in our body, mainly to important capillaries developed by exercise. Due to the efficient gas exchange in the lungs, fatigue would be reduced, benefiting not only the heart, but also the whole body. According to him, "Contrology exercises guard against unnecessary pounding or throbbing of your heart. [8]"

As demonstrated up until now, Pilates method offers several benefits to the physiological systems. In the neuroendocrine system, for instance, the harmony between the movements of the respiratory chain and the muscular chain provides balance to the sympathetic and parasympathetic nervous systems, which could reduce anxiety symptoms and wakefulness. According to some studies, exercises, when well applied and periodized, can increase the production of neurotransmitters associated with mood and well-being, such as serotonin, dopamine, and endorphin neuropeptides, classified as natural opioids [18].

The methodology developed by Pilates through seemingly simple exercises, such as "footwork" and respiratory maneuvers, demonstrates the importance of this work for the preservation of cardiac functions and prevention of cardiovascular diseases.

Chapter 18

RESPIRATORY SYSTEM: BREATHING PRINCIPLE APPLIED TO THE PILATES METHOD

The respiratory and cardiovascular systems are efficient in the transport of oxygen to and removal of carbon dioxide from all tissues.

There are two breathing processes: external respiration and internal respiration. External respiration involves the transport of gases from outside the body into the lungs and then into the bloodstream. Internal respiration begins when blood reaches the tissues. Both external respiration and internal respiration are linked to the cardiovascular system [19].

Respiratory efficiency is often responsible for the good performance of the circulatory system and for the control of cardiac functions.

Respiratory exercise training applied to the Pilates method requires a lot of practice and discipline from the student. With time, the student will acquire his/her own breathing rhythm and, consequently, higher respiratory efficiency and range of motion.

For beginners, respiration is seen as one of the most difficult principles of the method, and there exist many reasons why some people find it hard to discover their breathing rhythm. The most anxious students, for example, are more reluctant to the exercises. In many cases, some instructors end up overlooking this principle and pay more attention to the technique associated with the physical exercises. But this principle and all the others are important, as they are essential for the good performance of Pilates exercises. However, teaching respiratory movements demands more attention from the instructor, who plays a leading role in this process. Moreover, when students find the benefits of respiratory maneuvers and their breathing rhythm, the benefits are even larger, including reduction of anxiety (quite common in adults and elderly people, which can prevent or delay the use of medication), mastery of movements, and improved concentration, not only on exercises, but also on cognitive activities.

Hypertensive individuals need extra attention to the exercises. The initial procedure is to check blood pressure before the training sessions, with a weekly follow-up to determine the average blood pressure. In general, these students have a great deal of difficulty in performing forced expiration. In some exercises in which this maneuver is essential for carrying out the movements, students tend to have apneic episodes (for holding their breath), which can increase blood pressure. The position in which the exercises are performed also matters in the case of hypertensive individuals. In the lying position, blood pressure tends to increase and, therefore, it is recommendable to have students perform more intense and moderate exercises in the sitting or standing position. For hypotensive individuals, the lying position is beneficial, as it helps normalize the systolic and diastolic blood pressure.

All these aspects were observed by Pilates when he worked with his students. He carefully analyzed the poses depicted in the pictures and checked the difference in blood pressure in different positions (sitting, reclining, and lying). Quoting him, "This is done to relieve your heart from undue strain as well as to take advantage of the more normal (original) position of the visceral organs of your body when in such positions. Contrary to exercises performed in an upright position, those performed while you are in a recumbent position do not aggravate any possible undetected organic weakness."

Breathing in the Pilates method, when well applied and guided, provides a lot of benefits to practitioners. When we breathe slowly and expiration is longer than inspiration, cardiac rhythm and blood pressure decrease slightly. These respiratory movements demand full concentration from the student, taking him/her to a state of meditation, thereby balancing the sympathetic and parasympathetic systems.

In order to explain the methodological aspects of breathing to his students, Pilates relied on metaphors. He said: "To breathe correctly, you must completely exhale and inhale, always trying very hard to "squeeze" every atom of impure air from your lungs in much the same manner that you would wring every drop of water from a wet cloth. When you stand erect again, the lungs will automatically completely refill themselves with fresh air."

Pilates claimed that, besides the benefits for the respiratory and circulatory systems, complete exhalation and inhalation of air increased the activity of all muscles. He said that when the whole body is profusely charged with fresh air, revitalized blood reaches down the fingertips and toe tips, "similarly as the heat generated by a good head of steam in your boiler and properly distributed by your radiators is felt in every room in your house." For Pilates, people who failed to master the art of proper breathing were at a great disadvantage in relation to longevity. "Lazy breathing converts the lungs, figuratively speaking, into a cemetery for the deposition of diseased, dying, and dead germs as well as supplying an ideal haven for the multiplication of other harmful germs." [9]

The breathing technique in the Pilates method aims to increase the efficiency of expiratory pressure, which is reduced by several factors, such as postural deformity – observed, for instance, in hyperkyphosis, which decreases the distension of the lungs and of the chest wall – aging, and inactivity. We can therefore say that expiratory efficiency increases the gas exchange capacity, mainly residual air exchange, thereby maintaining the ideal pH in the lungs and preventing respiratory infections.

In the respiratory chain, the diaphragm is one of the major inspiratory muscles, being constantly recruited in Pilates respiratory movements, in addition to the transverse abdominal muscle, contributing to spinal column stability. Then, the main muscles involved in forced expiration are the abdominal muscles, which provide generalized pressure to the diaphragm.

During activation of respiratory work, there is the participation of groups of muscles that stay active, acting as stabilizers and helping with breathing.

Electromyographic studies show that the breathing movement technique, together with trunk flexion movement, is responsible for the largest activation of the transverse abdominal and internal oblique muscles [22].

We may say that, in Pilates exercises, there is an association between the respiratory chain and the kinetic chains and that both are responsible for the precision of movements and stability of the hip and of the spinal column.

In 2009, I carried out a study to evaluate respiratory functions in a group of elderly women with hyperkyphosis. The training was performed during seven months using basic-level exercises. The outcomes were quite satisfactory. There was an increase in maximal expiratory pressure in the group that practiced Pilates exercises.

In the study of Tinoco-Fernández et al. (2016), the practice of Pilates exercises for 10 consecutive weeks revealed a positive impact on cardiorespiratory parameters in healthy adults who did not practice sports or physical exercises on a regular basis [23].

At present, few studies have assessed respiratory functions in the Pilates method. I believe that future research with implementation of Pilates workout will corroborate its efficiency in these groups. The Pilates method will be regarded as a preventive and nonpharmacological option for several diseases, in addition to offering many benefits, such as improvement in posture, health, and well-being.

Chapter 19

NEUROMUSCULAR SYSTEM

Movement occurs through neuromuscular activity. The nervous system provides an electrical signal that induces muscle contraction. These systems (neural and muscular) work together, inducing normal and specific movements. It is possible to affirm that all functions in the human body are influenced by the nervous system. Nevertheless, in order for muscles to contract, they have to produce reserve energy (adenosine triphosphate – ATP) continuously, which means that the metabolic system is also responsible for muscle contraction and, therefore, for the physical activities and exercises we perform every day.

The physiological changes derived from physical training are specific to the type of physical preparation used. The structure and functioning of the muscle being exercised determine the type of muscle fiber and its importance to specific types of activities [19].

An individual's ability to perform an exercise is the cause, and the movement per se is the effect. It is paramount to control the cause to obtain a successful effect. Biomotor skills, which underlie the cause, are mostly genetically inherited. The genes we inherit determine which motor neurons will innervate our muscle fibers. After innervation, our muscle fibers differentiate themselves (become specialized) according to the type of neuron that stimulates them. Nonetheless, there is some evidence suggesting that endurance training and muscle inactivity could cause a deviation or changes in myosin isoforms (which characterizes the type of muscle fiber as fast- or slow-twitch). These modifications can result in moderate changes in the percentage of fast-twitch fibers (FTF). Furthermore, both in aging and inactivity, this type of fiber is largely debilitated compared with slow-twitch fibers (STF).

The human neuromuscular system reaches full maturation between the ages of 20 and 30 years. From the ages of 30 to 40 years, maximum force stays the same or decreases slightly. However, around the age of 60 years, maximal muscle strength decreases by 30 to 40%, which corresponds to the debilitation of FTF. Moreover, the consequences of constant muscle injuries are important as they often expedite and change the aging of muscle fibers.

Muscle injuries can also affect neuromuscular proprioception, causing functional damage rather than a structural one. The structure may be intact when observed by static evaluation, but probably shows dysfunctional movements.

The neuromuscular proprioception system can recognize the spatial location of the body, its position, and orientation. It represents the force exerted by the muscles and the position of each body part relative to the others without using vision. It may also be defined as control of movement. This type of "sense" allows maintaining balance, with interaction of muscle fibers that work to keep the body in its base of support, information on touch and on the vestibular system, located in the inner ear [24].

In the Pilates method, basic exercises are performed in order to deal with proprioception through the introduction of the principles of movement control and centering.

These exercises are moderate, with the use of strength by the activation of more motor units and, consequently, of more STF. Thus, according to the classification of the exercises, as intensity increases, FTF are recruited. The same recruitment pattern is followed during long activities (e.g., long-distance running) [19].

In general, STF are recruited more often than FTF. On average, most muscles are composed of nearly 50% of STF and 25% of FTF; the classification of the remaining fibers is still being investigated. The exact percentage of these types of fibers varies considerably among muscles and also among individuals.

Individual characteristics such as biotype can determine the dominant type of muscle fiber and the type of innervation. As an example, let us look at the biotypes of a marathoner and a sprinter. A marathoner is an ectomorph, i.e., slim with skinny calves, whereas the sprinter is a mesomorph, with fat calves and higher percentage of muscle mass. This analysis is subjective and may therefore be error-prone.

For a more objective and accurate analysis, some researchers apply an invasive technique, using a biopsy needle to collect a leg muscle sample. This method allows investigating and classifying muscle fibers by way of microscopic and biochemical analyses. The cost of this type of analysis is prohibitive nowadays, so it is used only for elite athletes. Thanks to these analyses, we learned that marathon world champions have 50 to 99% of STF in their gastrocnemius muscles, whereas sprinters have only 25% of STF in the same muscles. STF have high aerobic resistance and are particularly suitable for endurance and low-intensity activities [19].

Muscle fatigue is another factor that may change the recruitment pattern of muscle fibers. It may occur in several situations, especially when the muscles are subjected to an activity or exercise with maximum effort and short duration. Fatigue can alter muscle adaptations and thus modify the muscle fiber recruitment pattern. Hence, both control and stability would be reduced, mainly in the trunk and hip muscles. This imbalance could result in muscle spasm (intense contraction of the muscles), often causing acute pain. Rehabilitation with a physical therapist is indicated in these cases.

The Pilates method basically works with trunk and hip stabilization. This is achieved by recruiting STF, also known as red fibers. These fibers are in constant contraction. They remain active for several hours each day, usually for controlling posture. Recall that the recruitment of muscle fibers depends on the type of activity. For example, FTF are recruited in high-speed running and in maximal strength exercises. These fibers are less resistant and develop fatigue more quickly.

When a muscle shortens, the sliding of fibers past each other occurs less often at the onset of contraction. This activates important neural pathways that control muscle length during movement and postural adjustments.

The specificity of Pilates exercises is highly beneficial for the maintenance of posture and well-being. In addition to the benefits that are clearly evident for students and instructors, recent studies have suggested Pilates exercises can increase the production of antioxidant proteins, which are responsible for reducing free radicals, which cause the premature death of cells and, consequently, the intensification of aging.

Chapter 20

Control of Movement by the Muscles

If we compare our neural circuits with the circuits of a computer, we can see some similarity. Just as a machine has to be programmed to start operating, so does our neural system. The difference lies in processing time.

Precision of movement will be determined by the level of stimulation received and by favorable response conditions.

All movements produced by the musculoskeletal system are activated by the lower motor neurons, in the spinal cord and in the brainstem, which innervate directly the skeletal muscles.

The neural circuits in charge of controlling movement can be split into four different subsystems. They are totally interactive, each of them contributing in a unique fashion to motor control [24].

Before initiating the movement, we use a proactive and posture control feedback mechanism. The responses are pre-programmed and precede the first limb movements. For instance, in the contraction of the biceps (using some resistance), to ensure trunk stability, the contraction of the gastrocnemius muscle precedes that of the biceps [24].

As we can observe, the circuits of our body work together in harmony. The encephalon and the rest of the body are in constant communication, and both are responsible for maintaining or developing harmony.

The movement begins in the main motor neuron pathway that originates in the cortical frontal lobe and includes projections of the primary motor area and of neighboring premotor areas. These areas are responsible for planning and selecting movements, whereas the primary motor cortex is in charge of performing the movements. As discussed earlier, brainstem pathways organize the control of movement independently. Nevertheless, the projections of neurons in the brainstem and in the spinal cord are essential. This occurs mainly in fine and fractionated movements of the distal regions of the limbs, of the tongue and of the face, which are especially important in our daily activities.

Currently, neuroscientists have undertaken important studies on neuroplasticity, i.e., the capacity of neurons to create new connections in certain encephalic regions through external stimuli. Regardless of age or of neuronal integrity, physical exercises, when carefully guided, can stimulate neuroplasticity and, consequently, lead to significant outcomes, such as better quality of life and functional independence in patients with neurological disorders.

Recent studies have suggested that physical exercises also help improve overall cell functions of neurons and glial cells, activating growth factors both in the neurons and in the glial cells, thereby contributing to the development of new cells, in addition to improving brain functions.

The number of glial cells is 10 times larger than the number of neurons. These cells play important roles in the preservation of neurons. They have an efficient system for damage repair, in addition to the regulation and release of neurotransmitters.

These concepts support the assumption that Pilates physical exercises, when properly explained and implemented, may be useful for the treatment of degenerative diseases and for the rehabilitation of cognitive disorders [25].

Chapter 21

NEUROPLASTICITY AND PILATES EXERCISES

The Pilates method makes use of several resources, allowing for good outcomes as far as neuroplasticity is concerned. Apart from being indicated to improve movements and motor coordination, the method is very important in the rehabilitation of special cases.

The touching story of Siva Kalyan, an Australian boy of Indian origin, is a classic example. Siva had cerebral palsy caused by perinatal hypoxia. The motor cortex was the most affected region of the encephalon. Notwithstanding, his cognitive functions were preserved. After incessant attempts to treat Siva's neurological problems, his mother found out the benefits of the Pilates method, which was recommended by close relatives.

Since the method was very resourceful, providing good chances of meeting Siva's needs, Siva and his parents left for the USA and fixed their dwellings in Princeton (NJ). His parents entertained the hope of a better quality of life for their son, placing their faith in the Pilates method.

With time, several problems associated with Siva's condition began to emerge, such as muscle atrophy, ligamentous laxity (which caused scoliosis, hyperkyphosis, and rotation of the spinal column), among others, besides respiratory problems and chronic luxations. Before they moved to the USA, Siva's family had sought all kinds of treatment, but to no avail, until they heard of Anthony Rabara. Anthony Rabara had a degree in dance and had worked with Romana Kryzanowska for many years, gaining a lot of experience, which he could then use to treat Siva.

In 2000, Siva was 9 years old when Rabara began treating him with Pilates exercises. At the beginning, Siva was confined to a wheelchair and had to be supported by a belt, which delayed the aggravation of his scoliosis. After 5 years, Siva achieved surprising outcomes with the training sessions.

In 2007, Romana asked Rabara to present his results at the Pilates Conference in Las Vegas (USA). At the Conference, Siva was pushed in a wheelchair by his parents. Siva's grandfather had filmed several training sessions throughout the years. Rabara then shared the videos with the audience, showing the progress achieved with his work. After the presentation, Siva went to the Cadillac to demonstrate a series of intermediate exercises, with some modifications and adaptations. After the demonstration, much to everyone's surprise, Siva grabbed his pair of crutches and started walking. It was a touching moment for all those people at the event [26].

This case study and the recent clinical trials about degenerative diseases and cognitive disorders underscore the importance of devotion to and trust in the Pilates method, mainly among health professionals and physical educators.

Chapter 22

METABOLIC SYSTEM: BODY COMPOSITION

Lately, the incidence of overweight has increased alarmingly in all age groups and social strata, but mainly among children and adolescents. This problem has been observed since the early 1950s in industrialized countries. In 1954, *Life Magazine* published an article entitled: "The plague of overweight."

At that time, there was a deep concern with an obesity epidemics. Approximately 5 million Americans were considered to be obese and weighed at least 20% more than what was regarded as normal weight. As a result, mortality rate was higher. Another 20 million Americans were classified as overweight (10% above healthy weight). The consequences of these changes are a tendency towards developing metabolic syndrome, physical incapacitation, and complications during surgeries and during pregnancy. [27]

At present, the figures mentioned by Life magazine have increased even more dramatically: according to the latest studies, over one-third of U.S. adults (35.7%) and around 17% (or 12.5 million) of children and adolescents aged 2 to 19 years are overweight.

As with the USA, several other countries, both industrialized and developing, have had to cope with this serious public health problem.

It is common knowledge that modern man's lifestyle has influenced eating habits which, combined with a sedentary lifestyle, are not good for overall health.

In Brazil, the National Food and Nutrition Policy points out that obesity is one of the greatest challenges nowadays and its guidelines recommend continuing care of individuals who suffer from overweight and obesity.

According to the World Health Organization (WHO), obesity can be understood as a multifactorial condition triggered by a positive energy balance, which predisposes to fat accumulation, associated with risks for the development of metabolic syndrome. Among the causes for obesity, we have biological, historical, ecological, economic, social, cultural, and political factors [28].

There has been a long-standing vigorous debate about the emergence of diseases associated with weight gain. Among adults and elderly, obesity and overweight are the major cause of morbidity and mortality in both industrialized and developing countries.

Cardiovascular diseases stem from metabolic disorders whose influence necessitates further investigation. In this respect, it has been well established in the scientific literature and in clinical practice that metabolic syndrome is a cardiovascular risk factor, often related to central fat deposition, or central obesity, and insulin resistance [29].

Obesity is accompanied by an increase in the production of reactive oxygen species (ROS), either because of an imbalance in the clearance of ROS (which takes place at the intracellular level), or because of the larger production of oxidative stress. These effects could result from excessive calorie intake and from the saturation of the electron transport chain, as well as from the production of free radicals by cellular systems. As a consequence, some changes occur in the production of insulin or cytokines, which are characteristic of obesity [30].

Chapter 23

WHAT IS METABOLIC SYNDROME?

Metabolic syndrome is a complex metabolic disorder triggered by a dysfunction in homeostasis, also known as "civilization syndrome." It is related to carbohydrate, lipid, and protein metabolism, and to genetic programming and predisposition as well (Gottlieb MGV et al., 2008). Aside from these factors, sedentary lifestyle is also associated with the increased risk for development of this syndrome (PARK et al., 2003)

As pointed out by Park et al. (2003), the incidence and prevalence of metabolic syndrome increase with age, especially after the age of 60 years, both in men and women. According to the authors, the prevalence of this syndrome in the USA is around 23% in nonelderly individuals (male or female), rising to 43% in individuals aged over 60 years. Their study showed also that metabolic syndrome affected 4.6% of individuals with normal weight, 22.4% of overweight individuals, and 59.6% of obese individuals.

The standardization of diagnostic criteria for metabolic syndrome is hindered by ethnic groups with genetic variants and different cultural patterns [31, 32].

To overcome this problem, the International Diabetes Federation (IDF) has established a new set of criteria for use in both epidemiological studies and clinical practice worldwide. The aim is to identify those individuals with metabolic syndrome in order to elucidate the etiology of the syndrome and to focus on therapeutic strategies for reducing the risk for cardiovascular diseases. [33]

In recent years, the incidence of metabolic syndrome has increased substantially, and this has been extensively investigated to determine its etiopathogenicity and clinical management. Gottlieb et al. conducted a review of the main genetic, evolutionary, and nutritional aspects involved in the development of metabolic syndrome. The authors asserted that, as genes express its effects on phenotype by means of biochemical reactions, these effects depend on the chemical and physical media in which the reactions take place. Therefore, eating habits and lifestyle (especially physical activity), may be crucial for the development of metabolic disorders, as occurs with metabolic syndrome.

Table 1. Prevalence of metabolic syndrome according to the World Health Organization (WHO), European Group for the Study of Insulin Resistance (EGIR), and the National Cholesterol Education Program – Adult Treatment Panel III (NCEP ATP III)

	WHO	EGIR	NCEP ATP III
Australia	**≥ 30 years**	**> 24 years**	
Men	25.2	18.6	19.5
Women	16.7	13.3	17.2
France	**30-65 years**		
Men	23.0	16.4	10.0
Women	12.0	10.0	7.0
Mauritius	**> 24 years**		
Men	20.9	9.0	10.6
Women	17.6	10.2	14.7

Source: Alberti K.G.M.M. et al., 2009.

Chapter 24

THE ORIGIN OF METABOLIC SYNDROME

Human evolution studies demonstrate large morphological and physiological changes in the human body over time. The human brain went through remarkable changes in the evolutionary period.

Morphological studies on the skulls of the first hominids (e.g., *Homo habilis*, *Homo erectus*) and of Neanderthals show the structure of those skulls had gone through significant changes. The posterior region, known as posterior lobe, was longer, and so were the maxillary and mandibular bones. Thus, the anterior region (frontal lobe) was shorter. By looking at this body of evidence, we perceive the skull of primitive men went through changes because of survival needs and of modifications in their eating habits, such as the consumption of grains and fruits and the reduction in the intake of meat. This is reflected in the smaller size of maxillary and mandibular bones.

The neuroanatomical structure turned the modern man into an individual with superior reasoning ability with higher chances of survival.

However, ever since the Paleolithic age (50,000 BC to 1,000 BC), human genome has been virtually the same, i.e., the spontaneous mutation rate is low, around $1x10^{-5}$ to $1x10^{-6}$ for *Homo sapiens* (modern man). Currently, our diet differs markedly from that our genes were selected for. What has actually changed are the habits and lifestyle of the post-Industrial

Revolution man. In the Paleolithic age, men were basically hunters, collectors (collecting fruits and roots to complement the diet, a habit that was probably acquired from observing wild animals), and nomads (roaming from one place to another in search of food, because of environmental factors) [34].

Periods of hunger and thirst were often longer. It was at that time that energy-saving genes, as we know today, were selected. These genes store energy in the form of glycogen in the liver and in muscles during feeding.

The basic structure for physiological gene regulation was also selected at that time; a time at which physical activity was a need for survival.

We may say that nutrition and physical activity are the two most important environmental factors in the evolutionary process.

Nevertheless, genetics determines susceptibility to diseases, whereas environmental factors determine which genetically susceptible individual will be affected.

Changes throughout the human evolutionary history have affected the cellular metabolism, leading to the emergence of noncommunicable chronic diseases. Therefore, it is paramount to understand how these changes took place and their pathophysiological impact on the body in order to identify individuals who are more susceptible to noncommunicable chronic diseases and to devise strategies for their prevention [34].

Interesting genetic studies, more specifically in the areas of nutrigenetics and nutrigenomics, have been performed to investigate obesity. Nutrigenetics investigates the effects of genetic variability in relation to diets and diseases, whereas nutrigenomics assesses the influence of nutrients on genes and biological processes.

In other words, these studies evaluate the influence of genetic variability on nutrition, taking into account the metabolism of each individual. It is an important tool that facilitates the personalization of diets by specialized nutritionists.

Each individual responds differently to the diet and to the physical exercises. Some lose weight quickly; others take longer to obtain a satisfactory outcome.

So, it is essential that physical educators have enough knowledge of this area when prescribing physical activities and exercises.

Chapter 25

BODY COMPOSITION AND PILATES EXERCISES

There are several types of exercises and diets that promise losing weight quickly and efficiently. However, the results obtained with these exercises and diets last for a very short period of time and they could have irreversible consequences. Dissociations between body and mind can lead to the development of orthopedic, metabolic, and psychiatric diseases.

Recommendation of low-intensity and long aerobic activities, aimed at optimizing fat burn, is one of the strategies designed by health professionals, sometimes with unduly scientific evidence. According to the American College of Sports Medicine guidelines, pleasure and well-being should be a priority in any weight loss program, and physical activities and exercises have to be carefully selected for that purpose.

The association between exercises and suffering is probably one of the main off-putting aspects related to the practice of physical activity and proper exercising. Moreover, an inappropriate environment, which is competitive and focuses on immediate results, in addition to fast-paced music and standardized exercises, can prompt students to develop anxiety disorders. This is a very common sign in obese individuals, whose binge behaviors are often an attempt to eliminate anxiety. This makes students feel out of place and eventually quit the exercise practice.

As the Pilates method uses an educational approach, the exercises are performed in an environment that conveys calmness and introspection, making the students feel more confident and at ease.

It is known that working all muscles simultaneously and continuously through precise movements is the most efficient method for improving endurance and energy expenditure. The Pilates method was planned to work directly with the deepest muscles, thus allowing building a strong core, with no pain, as usually occurs in conventional exercises.

In the book *Pilates' Return to Life through Contrology*, Pilates showed his concern with overweight, underscoring that since man is not a hibernating creature, such excess of fat is a real detriment to him, imposing an unnecessarily heavy burden on his heart, liver, bladder, and other vitally important organs of his digestive system. Pilates then selected specific exercises for overweight individuals. Most times, he increased the number of repetitions and speed of the exercises to achieve larger energy expenditure. He used to say that a careful selection of specific Contrology exercises would allow for a good health status.

At present, scientific studies that evaluate overweight individuals subjected to Pilates exercises have shown significant results concerning changes in body composition, such as decrease of fat mass and increase of lean mass, in addition to changes in some components of metabolic syndrome, such as glucose, triglycerides, and waist circumference [35].

A systematic review of the effect of the Pilates method on risk factors for cardiometabolic diseases has pointed out the efficiency of exercises in reducing those components of metabolic syndrome. Approximately 86% of the studies included in this review revealed the efficacy of the Pilates method in the reduction of body and physiological components. It is common knowledge that these benefits, mainly the reduction in abdominal fat, waist-to-hip ratio, and blood pressure have a clinically important impact on the morbidity and mortality of cardiovascular diseases and cerebrovascular accident (stroke) [36].

These findings were also found in a study of adult women diagnosed with hyperkyphosis [14].

The results of these and other studies suggest that the energy expenditure and postural correction obtained through Pilates exercises may improve adipose tissue distribution through larger mobilization of the fat accumulated in the abdominal region.

This could also be related to the respiratory maneuvers carried out in the Pilates method, which require constant contraction of abdominal muscles in forced expiration, performed along with multidimensional and precise movements. To make these movements with higher precision it is necessary to use the concentration principle. This principle is quite efficient, as it leads the student into a state of meditation, balancing the sympathetic and parasympathetic systems.

These physiological changes obtained through the exercises are of utmost importance for homeostasis, especially of the endocrine, vascular, and neurological systems.

When planning an exercise regimen, it is important to observe the period for neural adaptation. During this period, the body programs itself for the correct performance of the exercises, improving the performance in more intense and longer exercises in the future.

Both intensity and number of exercises should be planned according to each student's needs. Basically, composition of muscle fibers and biological age determine the oxidative capacity of the muscles. This oxidative capacity is determined by the number of mitochondria and by the amount of oxidative enzymes. This metabolism depends chiefly on adequate oxygen supply. A longer training time is therefore important so that proper physical condition can be acquired.

Moderate exercises should be indicated for weight loss and for the balance between the increase in free radicals and the production of endogenous antioxidants [35]. Intense exercises, when done inappropriately, cause imbalance to these systems, producing early cell death and, consequently, hastening the aging process.

Hence, the Pilates method can be efficient if the exercise regimen is well planned with the aim of providing physical conditioning for future periodization of aerobic endurance exercises.

Chapter 26

PILATES METHOD: FLEXIBILITY AND STRETCHING

Flexibility and stretching can be distinguished based on their methodological and physiological concepts. Stretching depends on different muscle functions, such as direction of muscle fibers, angles at which the exercises are performed, in addition to factors that could restrict movements. Flexibility is the outcome of this work, which allows range of motion by way of joint movements, following the normal pattern of the muscles. Many are the factors that may hinder flexibility, among which we can cite the shape of joint surfaces, bone formation, adhesions, contractures, and soft tissue scarring, besides contractile components such as ligaments, tendons, and fascial stiffness [37]. I believe the determining factors for lack of flexibility or for hypermobility are the shapes of joint and bone surfaces, which are related to the student's individual characteristics, including sex, race, and genetic code. In this case, we may consider these factors to be irreversible and likely to restrict or increase flexibility.

Hypermobility, in some cases, is classified as a joint hypermobility syndrome, as observed among contortionists who perform movements at closed angles with twists. Studies indicate a prevalence of 5 to 15% of hypermobility in women, especially in Asian ones. However, this prevalence decreases with age, but it can increase with stretching exercises. [37]

Differently from what most people think, joint hypermobility is not beneficial. Over time, it may cause several musculoskeletal disorders. Spontaneous arthroses are more frequent, mainly in lower limbs and in the spinal column, producing painful joint fatigue and wear. Pain becomes more intense during climate changes and at the onset of each menstrual cycle.

Hypermobility declines over the years, but pain persists. In some cases, there are signs of spondylolisthesis and orthoarthrosis, in addition to chronic and acute pain.

People with muscle, joint, and fascial stiffness are also prone to different types of injuries, chiefly to the hip and to the spinal column, including herniated discs. In general, men have larger stiffness or the so-called muscle shortening. Nevertheless, specific stretching exercises have contributed a lot to significantly reducing this stiffness and increasing the joint angle.

Due to aging and inactivity, these conditions become worse, since numerous changes occur in the body, especially in the musculoskeletal, endocrine, and vascular systems [19].

In the musculoskeletal system, aside from the age-associated wear, such as reduction of distal space and of joints in general, there is also a decrease in elastin production and an increase in collagen production. Consequently, fascial stiffness develops, acting as a protective system.

For all the reasons described above, it is important to have a method with exercises that can improve flexibility, strength, and endurance in all population groups, but mainly in elderly people.

Numerous studies have demonstrated that Pilates exercises, primarily those performed on apparatuses, could be safe and beneficial, improving these physical parameters and posture as well. The spring system of the Pilates apparatuses is an excellent resource for working with flexibility. Apart from improving strength and endurance, the system provides progressive assistance during stretching and flexibility exercises, protecting the muscles and the joints from any injuries. Flexibility exercises are recommended for two basic reasons: as preparation for the activity, facilitating the performance of the exercises, and as a means to reduce the probability of injury during the exercises.

In 2009, I conducted a study with ladies with a mean age of 60 years who had been diagnosed with hyperkyphosis. My objective was to assess changes in posture and in flexibility before and after a Pilates exercise regimen. The findings indicate significant improvement in posture, with an 8° reduction in hyperkyphosis, and also an increase in flexibility, evaluated at all joint angles. [14] This study corroborates data presented by other studies, in which Pilates exercises also helped improve flexibility.

Currently, physical assessment relies on different types of devices for evaluating flexibility. Measurements are not a precise standardized procedure with a well-established normative test. These devices, even though they are not standardized, are important for the design of a scientific study and for periodization of a specific training program, as in the case of professional athletes and dancers. Regardless of these resources, however, visual assessment performed in the classroom by the instructor is crucial for the planning of training sessions, ensuring their safety and efficiency. This assessment, along with posture evaluation (e.g., pictures) at different angles and positions, may be useful for a future comparative analysis (before and after) to confirm the efficacy of Pilates exercises.

Preserving joint mobility through Pilates flexibility exercises prevents any muscle chain from restricting broader and more complex movements. These exercises, when applied and performed correctly and objectively, promote harmony between agonist and antagonist muscles, rendering the movements more pleasant and fluid. To achieve that, in addition to the application of Pilates exercise techniques, some materials can be used to facilitate alignment and the performance of educational exercises aimed at preparing the body for more complex exercises.

There are several techniques that deal with flexibility, but the Pilates method, according to scientific evidence, is safer and alleviates muscle pain, especially low back pain.

Recall that a shortened muscle, in many cases, is not synonymous with a strong and resistant muscle, and neither would be a muscle, whose stretching exceeds normal standards. That is why endurance and muscle strength exercises should be accompanied by exercises targeted at developing or maintaining flexibility. Therefore, we may say that good posture is closely related to good flexibility.

PART 2

Chapter 27

AGING

Aging is usually defined as a process of progressive loss of functions, followed by infertility, morphofunctional changes (physiological, biochemical, and psychological), and finally by death, an event that is sure to come with advanced age.

This definition, for several people, especially for the younger ones, seems to be a faraway reality that marks the end of life. This is so because we tend to see only the negative aspects of aging and forget that a healthy and active aging process is a consequence of the lifestyle we chose to lead in all stages of life, starting *in utero*.

Biologically speaking, we begin to age during the cell divisions that take place at conception. Until we reach reproductive maturity, there will be molecular repair mechanisms, which will decrease over time.

How fast one ages depends on genetic and environmental factors. According to the genetic evolution theory, the specific genes that could accelerate or delay aging remain to be known.

Recent animal studies reveal that longevity can be extended by genetic mutation. It has been observed that genetic mutations in certain receptors and signaling proteins substantially increase longevity in mutant strains of worms, flies, and mice, indicating that genetic regulation mechanisms affect aging and longevity [38]. However, human aging theory studies demonstrate that genetic factors account for 30 to 40% of the aging process, whereas environmental factors represent 60 to 70%. This could mean that we have a chance of more than 60% to invest in a healthy life in all stages of our development, increasing our prospects of having an active and preeminent aging process.

Both healthy and unhealthy lifestyles are characterized by several variables. Sedentary lifestyle, inappropriate diet, smoking, drinking, and environmental pollution top the list of factors that speed up aging. All of these variables are relevant as they predispose to noncommunicable chronic diseases, such as cardiovascular diseases, diabetes, chronic respiratory diseases, and cancer [35].

Studies also reveal that maternal diet genetically programs embryonic or fetal cells. Thus, when the diet is poor and dysfunctional, it will be a risk factor for the development of chronic diseases in adult life, mainly cardiovascular diseases. Nevertheless, this process can be reversed later by changes in eating habits and by the regular practice of physical exercises.

Research indicates that these behaviors could help "silence" the genes that were programmed or activate the genes known as "survival genes," which are related to regular physical activities and to a sensible diet [39].

Aging, in many cases, results from the somatization of damage inflicted on the body. The biological processes inherent to aging are multifactorial and set a time limit to life, varying among individuals.

While longevity represents an improvement in human evolutionary processes, cognitive changes associated with aging are more and more prevalent in several industrialized countries.

We hope that, with the major breakthrough in genomics, there will be enough room for the development and testing of evolutionary theories, which explain the effects of stochastic and genetic factors on our body that will possibly affect future generations.

Chapter 28

BIOLOGICAL AGING

As Robin Holliday puts it, we age because we evolve from beings that also age. We age because our developed body structure is incompatible with indefinite survival. We age because our different mechanisms of maintenance cannot preserve this structure and the normal functions of cells and tissues. As human beings, we live longest because we evolved into a lifestyle with low annual mortality rates. That allowed more resources to be invested in maintenance compared to fewer resources in reproduction. Conversely, those species that live in a high-risk environment will only survive by investing more heavily in reproduction, with fewer resources allocated to maintenance [40].

The evolution of aging was initially explained by the idea that senescence is programmed to limit population size or accelerate the number of reproductions, helping organisms adapt to environmental changes [41].

In nature, biological aging differs depending on the species. This process depends on several factors that could hasten or slow down senescence (natural aging at the cell level).

Over the years, all cells in the human body senesce, that is, they lose their proliferative capacity after a given number of cell divisions.

There is scant evidence that senescence significantly contributes to mortality. Natural death, as opposed to the deaths that occur in protected populations, is higher because of the extrinsic environmental risks, which include infections, starvation, excessive cold, excessive sun exposure, physical stress, and emotional stress [41].

Notably, at the present time, these situations are observed in extremely poor countries, such as Sierra Leone (West Africa), where life expectancy at birth is globally the lowest: 32.4 years for men and 35.7 years for women [42].

In nature, as a general rule, wild animals do not live long enough to experience aging. Even in species in which senescence contributes to natural death (large mammals and some long-lived birds), any hypothesis for accelerated aging would be disadvantageous to the species [39].

Growing evidence suggests that cellular senescence and organic aging are antagonistic pleiotropic manifestations (multiple effects of one gene) of evolutionary pressures to prevent malignant transformation of diseases. In other words, aging could be the price we pay for warding off cancer. The good paradox could be that the maximum living potential of human beings may have been attained, due partly to our aging capacity [43].

Normal aging in humans involves inexorable and universal biological changes that are characteristic of the aging process, namely menopause, gray hair, wrinkles, and loss of renal function, among others. However, in usual aging, besides these biological changes, there is an increase in the prevalence of noncommunicable chronic diseases. These diseases result from the accumulation of damage throughout life, in addition to genetic factors, unhealthy eating habits, and sedentary lifestyle [44].

Many theories exist about the aging process. These theories are not clearly defined and necessitate further investigation, especially in studies with different groups in terms of lifestyle, climate changes, and environmental changes.

Several scholars have sought to use new theories to determine the main causes of aging in distinct populations. According to Troen, theories of aging can be split into two general categories: stochastic and genetic. The combination of stochastic and genetic factors may speed up or slow down the aging process [43].

The stochastic theory is related to random environmental events that lead to the accumulation of damage to the body, resulting in a progressive physiological decline. Stochastic factors, when in excess, are believed to accelerate aging, contributing towards the development of noncommunicable chronic diseases [44].

In the stochastic theory, several specific theories of aging stand out, including those of oxidative stress, somatic mutation, mitochondrial DNA damage, error catastrophe, DNA repair, protein modification, among others that are in the process of being investigated.

These theories deal with environmental phenomena that may change homeostasis, i.e., they can also alter our genes and therefore compromise future generations. On the other hand, a young body is capable of repairing damage at a higher speed and more efficiently, just as a system for the removal of altered proteins and other agents. In an old body, this process is compromised, contributing to the progressive accumulation of damage and to inefficient DNA repair. Hence, aging is the outcome of these environmental phenomena rather than their cause.

Important studies with accurate assessments of genetic and environmental influences on different populations have been underway. These studies help predict the future emergence (or not) of diseases, encompassing many fields of the health area, gathering information for well-reasoned recommendations with regard to disease prevention.

As an example, we have relevant studies that could contribute to the efficacy and safety in medication use, especially when treating elderly people.

Pharmacogenetics and/or pharmacogenomics is the study of genetic influences on drug responses. Pharmacogenetics focuses on the effects of isolated genes, whereas pharmacogenomics explores simultaneously several genes and their interactions. These subfields of clinical pharmacology seek to optimize medical care through personalized treatment, taking into account the different genetic characteristics of individuals. More specifically, they aim to identify genes that: (A) predispose to diseases; (B) modulate drug responses; (C) affect the pharmacokinetics and pharmacodynamics of medications, and (D) are associated with adverse drug reactions [17].

Besides these important studies, as previously mentioned in other chapters, nutrigenetics and nutrigenomics are important tools for a personalized nutritional guidance, with the aim of preventing and treating severe and progressive diseases.

Given that the research into chronic diseases is significantly complex, nutrigenomic studies are the best option to elucidate molecular processes that keep the body healthy and prevent the development of diseases [45].

Analyses of genome provide complete genetic information (DNA and RNA). However, to obtain more specific information, large-scale studies on protein expression in different tissues and body fluids are being conducted. Recent methodological advancements in this area have opened up new opportunities for obtaining relevant information on normal and abnormal processes that take place in the human body. [46] As with the syndromes that accelerate aging, Werner syndrome makes individuals age 5 to 10 times more quickly than an otherwise healthy person. The diagnosis is made, on average, at the age of 36 years. Nevertheless, as this is a rare syndrome, the diagnosis may be hindered or delayed. The average life expectancy is 46 years, and the major causes of death include severe diseases such as cancer, cerebrovascular accident, and acute myocardial infarction [47].

Recent data on the prevalence of this syndrome indicate countries with founder mutations, as in the Japanese population, with an estimate of 1/167,000 cases, and in Sardinia (Italy), with an estimate of 1/120,000 cases.

The Hutchinson-Gilford progeria syndrome is extremely rare and manifests itself in the first years of life. This syndrome affects 1 to 8 million inhabitants (live births) around the world. Its prevalence is higher among Caucasian men and can be observed in 97% of 150 cases described in the literature [48]. In this syndrome, the rate of aging is accelerated up to sevenfold. Those children who have this syndrome have a very low life expectancy, living on average up to the age of 13 to 14 years, and eventually die from aging-related diseases, such as myocardial infarction or congestive heart failure [48].

Therefore, genetic studies on aging with healthy individuals have allowed determining the genes implicated in the development of age-associated diseases, but not the specific genes responsible for normal aging.

Among numerous genetic theories, we have the telomere shortening theory, also referred to as the "biological clock" syndrome. It is regarded as a biological marker of aging, but further evidence is lacking [49].

Telomeres are nucleoprotein structures that cap the ends of chromosomes, preserving their stability and integrity. Many factors are involved in this dynamics, but they have not been fully elucidated yet.

Numerous studies have related telomere shortening and several conditions associated with aging, such as chronic diseases, sedentary lifestyle, and poor habits in general (smoking, drinking, overeating) [49].

The neuroendocrine theory is considered, amongst other genetic theories, to be the most relevant one. It determines the initial hallmark of the aging process. According to this theory, aging is the result of the reduction in the levels of several hormones on the hypothalamic-pituitary-adrenal axis that control the reproductive and metabolic systems. Hypothalamic activity depends on the expression of specific genes that manifest themselves at the end of the reproductive period.

In addition to the natural aging process that occurs around the menopause (when the reproductive period ends), specific and multifactorial alterations arise, which favor weight gain and the development or aggravation of obesity. In women, both chronological age and ovarian aging contribute to the increase in waist circumference, in fat mass, and in loss of muscle mass [50]. These hormonal changes, combined with sedentary lifestyle and a dysfunctional diet, may lead to the development of several cardiometabolic diseases. [35]

Last but not least, still in the field of genetic theories, we have the immunological theory. It is widely known that aging implies the reduction of body defenses owing to the lower number of cells in charge of eliminating pathogens. However, the mechanism that controls the cell cycle can be modified by stochastic factors, which override gene regulation factors associated with the aging process.

For this reason, it is difficult to know how the genes responsible for aging can accelerate or keep the state of balance. When homeostasis is lost, there is a decrease in the adaptability to stochastic aggressive events and, consequently, higher susceptibility to diseases [34].

It is commonly knowledge that longevity determinants are multifactorial and involve complex processes, most of which are still not fully understood. In recent years, however, there has been a significant advance in molecular biology studies, which help elucidate some of the major molecular mechanisms that influence aging and longevity.

We highlight many of the major findings and their possible clinical implications. Most of the intracellular factors associated with aging are still being investigated, such as research into sirtuins (enzymes in charge of binding and silencing cell longevity genes) and also insulin and insulin-like growth factor (marker of prostate cancer development). These genes are found on interconnected pathways.

Sirtuins are activated by resveratrol, a compound originally isolated from red wine, which is popularly known to increase longevity. In mice, resveratrol slows down some aspects of aging, including cognitive processes [38]. However, a study in which these and other genes were manipulated in animal models revealed that the useful life of these animals may either increase or decrease [51].

Kappeler (2005) conducted a study with transgenic mice and noticed the migration of several genes that eventually increased the useful life of these animals and observed that these genes are associated with a decrease in the secretion of growth hormone (GH) and with its main IGF-1 effector. The study of such transgenic mutants, combined with the well-known effect of calorie restriction on aging, allows the determination of common mechanisms for the regulation of the useful life of mammals [52].

Kendel pointed out that calorie restriction might act upon the insulin pathway through genes, with participation of sirtuins [38].

Molecular genetics studies of long-lived individuals have identified several potential candidate genes linked to long life. It is too early to confirm these findings, though. In-depth investigations of genomic associations are needed for the collection of accurate information.

Despite the existence of new biomarkers of aging and health, and also of telomere dysfunction, advances in genetics and in molecular biology require interdisciplinary approaches for the attainment of healthy and active aging [51].

There are ongoing interesting studies in the field of genetics and neuroscience that could revolutionize the preventive and clinical treatments of chronic diseases.

Optogenetics is a biological technique that involves the use of light for the control of gene expression. It allows assessing the behavior and the neural circuits in specific cells. The technique consists in controlling genetically modified neurons through light at specific wavelengths [53]. Karl Deisseroth was the first scientist to research and develop this technique in living animals. Ever since, several fields of research have expressed interest in applying this nonpharmacological and noninvasive method, considered by many researchers to be relevant and auspicious.

Optogenetics can be used to manipulate neural tissue by depolarization or hyperpolarization of encoded neurons and to monitor the activation of genetically encoded voltage-sensitive fluorescent proteins. This allows tracking down stimuli, enabling the noninvasive identification of intracerebral circuits. In addition, this technique permits mapping out altered circuits, which is of great value in neurological and psychiatric evaluations and applications.

Animal models have demonstrated that this type of intervention may be applied to humans in the treatment of several aging-associated diseases, such as behavioral and degenerative diseases, including cognitive and memory dysfunction, depression, Parkinson's disease, epilepsy, and Alzheimer's disease, among others. These findings and those of many studies on nonpharmacological treatment of noncommunicable chronic diseases are consistent with the adoption of preventive measures by several countries, with the aim of rationalizing medication use and minimizing its consequences on the health of elderly patients, in addition to encouraging the formation of healthy habits and changes in lifestyle, especially with respect to the practice of physical activities and exercises, combined with a diet that includes antioxidant-rich foods.

The 2008 Physical Activity Guidelines for Americans recommend that elderly individuals should be mindful of their limiting chronic conditions and be as physically active as their abilities and conditions allow. Inactivity should be avoided for achievement of healthy aging.

Chapter 29

USUAL AGING

In recent years, many industrialized and developing countries have had to cope with the aging of their populations. And the rise in life expectancy has become a global concern for it boosts economic and social demands.

While there is evidence that older people are living longer, especially in high-income countries, the quality of these additional years is unclear. Research results are very inconsistent, both at the national and international levels. In addition, the trends within the different subgroups of a population may vary widely [54].

Geriatrics and gerontology play an important role in the aging process, seeking to ensure a better quality of life for this population. According to Muriguchi, life expectancy at birth refers to the number of years an individual is expected to live, whereas healthy life expectancy is the number of years of life expected to be lived in full health [42].

Life expectancy in African and high-income countries is incredibly unequal. Inequality in life expectancy at birth and in healthy life expectancy may exceed 53 and 50 years, respectively, especially in the poorest African countries. The main reason for this inequality is the lack of control of communicable diseases such as malaria and HIV and the lack of resources allocated to basic healthcare [54].

In higher income countries, the major concern today is with noncommunicable chronic diseases, which pose a threat to healthy life expectancy. In Japan, for instance, life expectancy at birth is 85.3 years and healthy life expectancy is 77.7 years for women, with a difference of 7.6 years. This is the national average; however, healthy life expectancy is higher in certain regions, as in Okinawa, known as the Island of Centenarians.

A discussion on the development of noncommunicable chronic diseases in elderly people has been held for approximately three decades, focusing mainly on genetic and metabolic factors and on lifestyle (especially with respect to physical activity and diet). The discussion and the scientific studies associated with it are of great relevance to public health, since cardiovascular diseases are the main cause of morbidity and mortality in many countries [55].

It is possible to say that usual aging is related to an unhealthy lifestyle, including smoking and drinking habits as well as the consumption of industrialized foods and a sedentary behavior. In addition to the normal biological changes associated with aging, in usual aging there is a progressive loss of functionality and decreased response to stress. Lifelong accumulation of such damage can cause changes in gene expression, silencing some genes related to health, or activating those related to diseases [39].

The biological and cellular mechanisms involved in the aging process are not fully understood. Complex interrelated factors participate in the process, including stress-induced oxidative enzymes, DNA damage, instability of mitochondrial and nuclear genomes, chronic noninfectious inflammation caused by increased production of adipocytokines and cytokines, changes in fatty acid metabolism, including excessive release of free fatty acids into the plasma, insulin resistance, accumulation of metabolic end products, such as glycation and advanced oxidation protein products that interfere with normal cell functions [57].

Chapter 30

CHRONIC DISEASES AND OXIDATIVE STRESS

It is common knowledge that scientific breakthroughs in the control of communicable diseases have contributed significantly to the decline in mortality rate in many countries, especially in industrialized countries. However, noncommunicable chronic diseases are the major concern at the moment, as they affect all social classes, all age groups, especially the elderly, and both sexes.

The incidence and prevalence of diseases are higher among the elderly, who are affected by cardiovascular diseases, cancer, dementia, osteoporosis, and metabolic syndrome, the latter of which includes a series of cardiovascular risk factors [59].

Noncommunicable chronic diseases (NCDs) are the leading cause of premature death and of loss of quality of life, imposing severe restrictions on daily activities. Of the 57 million deaths in the world in 2008, 36 million (63%) were due to NCDs, especially cardiovascular diseases, diabetes, cancer, and chronic obstructive pulmonary disease (COPD).

More than 80% of deaths caused by NCDs occur in low- or middle-income countries, and 29% of those who die are aged less than 60 years. In high-income countries, premature deaths account for only 13% [37].

The mechanisms that underlie the pathogenesis of NCDs consist mainly of modifications in the oxidative metabolism. Approximately 5% of the oxygen consumed via the oxidative metabolism is not used in the mitochondrial cycles that produce energy for the whole body [57]. Thus, surplus oxygen tends to lose two electrons from its outermost orbital, producing free radicals.

The oxidative stress theory, also called free radical theory of aging, is one of the most widely accepted explanations for the aging process. The theory postulates that increased levels of reactive oxygen species (ROS) lead to functional changes, to pathological conditions, and to other clinically observable signs of aging, and eventually to death [59].

Several experimental models have been designed to verify the effects of oxidative stress on the development of cardiometabolic diseases. Some animal studies have shown that oxidative stress increases insulin resistance and adiposity [60].

However, the production of free radicals under normal conditions is a continuous physiological pathway that performs several essential functions, allowing for optimal functioning of the cell system, which includes mediation of electron transfer in various biochemical reactions, ATP production, immunological processes, gene activation and regulation, and egg fertilization [60].

Nevertheless, the overproduction of ROS can lead to oxidative damage and cause oxidative stress – an imbalance between ROS production and antioxidant activities. Therefore, the overproduction of ROS could indicate a change in the endogenous antioxidant defense system, including enzymatic and non-enzymatic antioxidants, leading to stress-sensitive signaling pathways and to the development of pathological conditions [62].

The enzymatic defense system produces enzymes that are found both in the cytoplasm and in the mitochondria, and depend on cofactors that may differ according to these cellular compartments (cytoplasm and mitochondrion). For example, superoxide dismutase (SOD), found in the mitochondrion, requires manganese as a cofactor (SOD-Mn). This enzyme is very important for the survival and maintenance of the mitochondrion.

Studies have shown that moderate physical exercise and regular physical activity significantly increase the production of SOD-Mn in the mitochondria, as well as of other enzymes that are crucial for homeostasis.

Therefore, the increase in the production of free radicals from intense physical exercise may exceed the capacity of antioxidant defense systems and cause oxidative stress. Both positive and negative effects of ROS production on sports performance are taken into consideration [63].

Thus, the inefficient control of ROS production by this defense system is particularly related to sedentary lifestyle and to excessive training with irregular and intense exercises, not only increasing ROS production, but also leading to irreversible mitochondrial DNA damage.

The damaged mitochondria can trigger a cellular energy crisis, causing tissues to senesce and age. The accumulation of such damage decreases the cell's ability to generate ATP, resulting in a gradual loss of energy, followed by a decrease in the number of mitochondria per cell, compromising energy production efficiency for the remaining mitochondria [59].

During the aging process, both men and women have a poor antioxidant defense mechanism, with a consequent increase in ROS levels. In menopausal women, low estrogen production causes hypertriglyceridemia, hypercholesterolemia, and hyperlipoproteinemia, and the resulting oxidation prompts the accumulation of free radicals in the cells, which eventually increases oxidative stress [59]. Postmenopausal women exhibit high levels of leptin and larger waist circumference, which are important predictors of insulin resistance [64].

Leptin is a protein hormone produced in adipose tissue. Its production involves various physiological processes (e.g., reproduction) and relies on its own receptors. Physiological mechanisms linked to the synthesis and secretion of leptin, such as receptor binding, appetite regulation, and energy expenditure, are complex variables that have not been fully elucidated yet and that involve numerous hormones and neurotransmitters [66]. In healthy subjects, leptin concentration is <10 ng/mL, and in obese patients it ranges from 10 to 100 ng/mL. Studies suggest that leptin may increase oxidative stress by induction and interaction between superoxide (O2) and nitric oxide (NO), enhancing the activity of the antioxidant enzyme through enzymes such as SOD and GSH-px.

The imbalance between oxidants and antioxidants makes proteins more vulnerable to oxidation and to the formation of undesirable oxidation products. These products are called oxidative markers and are usually investigated in individuals with metabolic disorders, such as type 2 diabetes mellitus, hypertriglyceridemia, and low levels of high-density lipoprotein (HDL), in addition to other problems such as hypertension and high LDL levels [66, 67].

Important studies are currently being made on various types of oxidative markers, which result from end products of oxidative stress and may affect normal physiological activities. As an example, we can cite ischemia-modified albumin (IMA). Changes in serum albumin have been evaluated as a possible biochemical marker of cardiac ischemia.

According to Gottlieb et al., abnormal IMA levels are not present only in acute biological conditions, such as myocardial infarction, but also in microenvironments that could increase tissue hypoxia. In their study, patients with metabolic syndrome had higher levels of IMA, which could be an important subclinical marker of poor peripheral oxygenation and of a low-grade inflammatory process. In patients with hypercholesterolemia and diabetes, IMA levels were higher than in healthy individuals. This marker is frequently detected in patients with hyperglycemia. Hyperglycemia and inflammation reduce the ability of albumin to bind to cobalt, resulting in higher levels of IMA and C-reactive protein.

Ferric reducing ability of plasma (FRAP) is another important marker. It consists of a newly developed enzyme assay to directly test total antioxidant power. This assay investigates the relationship between antioxidant status, dietary habits, and risk of disease [68]. It is accurate enough to assess the bioavailability of antioxidants in dietary agents, helping monitor longitudinal changes in antioxidant status associated with an increase in the intake of dietary antioxidants, and to investigate the effects of the disease on the antioxidant status [68]. This assay is used clinically and shows considerable reduction in plasma iron in the antioxidant defense system.

Chapter 31

DIETARY (NON-ENZYMATIC) ANTIOXIDANT DEFENSE SYSTEM

The non-enzymatic defense system consists of food compounds with antioxidant properties available from many foods such as vegetables, fruits, grains, and teas.

Aside from nutritional characteristics, a diet contains elements with antioxidant properties. Morales-Gonzáles detected vitamins C, E, D, and A, some amino acids, flavonoids, and some trace elements in his study. All of these antioxidant elements are an adjuvant alternative for the treatment and prevention of chronic degenerative diseases, which have very high morbidity and mortality rates [69].

Several studies have claimed that a diet with certain groups of foods or nutrients may decrease the incidence of metabolic syndrome, improving its prevention and prognosis [70].

Epidemiological studies suggest that these foods can reduce the risk of development of noncommunicable chronic diseases, such as cancer, cardiovascular diseases, metabolic disorders, neurodegenerative diseases, and inflammatory conditions [71].

There is evidence that a broad array of bioactive compounds with extremely variable chemical structure and biological functions could have beneficial effects on human health. Flavonoids, which were recognized in several studies in the last decade as having antioxidant, anticarcinogenic, anti-inflammatory, antithrombotic, hypolipidemic, and antidiabetic effects, are among the most widely studied bioactive substances to date. They also have antibacterial and antiviral activities, which allow preventing and treating various diseases, especially cardiovascular diseases [72].

Flavonoids belong to the group of phenolic compounds, also called polyphenols, and are widely available in foods of plant origin that make up the human diet. In plants, they are in charge of essential functions such as pigmentation, growth, reproduction, and resistance to pathogens. The main sources of flavonoids are citrus fruits (lemon, orange, tangerine, grape, and apple), vegetables such as onions, tomatoes, and broccoli, and beverages such as wine, grape juice, and teas [72].

Several epidemiological studies have shown an inverse relationship between flavonoid consumption and the occurrence of cardiovascular diseases, and when ingested on a daily basis, these substances can help prevent chronic diseases. [73] Flavonoids act by relaxing the smooth muscles of the cardiovascular system, thus contributing to lowering blood pressure and improving overall circulation. Due to their antioxidant properties, they also prevent the oxidation of LDL cholesterol, responsible for the formation of atheromatous plaques, which increase the risk of thrombosis. [74]

Currently, in the field of functional food research, *Camellia sinensis* (green tea) has been widely investigated due to its specific flavonoid content, which provides it with numerous therapeutic properties. Its leaves are used for the production of various types of teas, including catechin-rich green tea, which is considered to have a potent preventive effect against cardiovascular diseases and other chronic diseases. [74] The chemical composition of green tea includes several classes of phenolic compounds such as flavans, flavonols, and phenolic acids, as well as caffeine, pigments, carbohydrates (5%), amino acids, and some micronutrients such as vitamins B, E, C and minerals like calcium, magnesium, zinc, potassium, and iron [75].

The study conducted by Junges (2016) on the effects of Pilates exercises and on supplementation with *Camellia sinensis* extract (CSE) revealed that such supplementation among sedentary individuals has a negligible effect on the diagnostic criteria for metabolic syndrome and on body composition. However, CSE when used in conjunction with moderate Pilates exercises produces greater effect, mainly on blood glucose and triglyceride levels and on waist circumference. As pointed out in the literature, when these parameters are increased, they serve as criteria for the diagnosis of several entities in studies on the prevalence, incidence, treatment, and prevention of metabolic syndrome [35].

In metabolic syndrome, there is usually an increase in fat mass and body fat percentage, but body weight apparently does not correlate with the amount of muscle mass. In some cases, this may indicate the presence of another progressive geriatric syndrome known as sarcopenia.

Chapter 32

Sarcopenia

Inactive aging, in addition to causing progressive loss of muscle and bone mass, imposing several limitations on the musculoskeletal system, weakens the main physiological systems (cardiovascular, respiratory, immune, and nervous systems) and increases the risk for the development of psychiatric disorders such as depression, cognitive impairment, and anxiety.

Depression is considered a common geriatric syndrome among inactive elderly individuals. However, in several cases, its symptoms are not identified, which leads to inadequate treatment. Many studies on institutionalized elderly patients with depression show some association between loss of muscle mass and depression. In recent years, sarcopenia (loss of muscle mass) has been increasingly described by several authors who investigate aging.

The term "sarcopenia" was proposed by Irwin Rosenberg in 1989 and is now widely accepted to describe the constant involuntary loss of skeletal muscle mass associated with aging. [76] Sarcopenia was defined by Irwin Rosenberg as loss of skeletal muscle mass and strength that occurs with age. Nevertheless, no widely accepted definition of sarcopenia that is appropriate for use in research and clinical practice has been provided so far [76].

It is common knowledge that the causes are complex and multifactorial, including neural degeneration, quality and quantity of muscle fibers, and decrease in the concentration of hormones that play an important role in cell metabolism. The consequences of these changes are loss of muscle strength and of endurance, as well as increases in free radical production and changes in balance and in posture. This frailty makes elderly people vulnerable to adverse events, including difficulty in performing basic instrumental activities, predisposition to osteoporosis, risk of falls, longer hospital stays, delayed return to daily activities, and eventually death.

Therefore, the importance of understanding the true prevalence of sarcopenia should be underscored in order to design effective preventive strategies [77].

The European Working Group on Sarcopenia in Older People (EWGSOP) provided a definition for clinical practice and a consensus diagnosis of age-related sarcopenia. For the diagnosis of sarcopenia, the EWGSOP recommends evaluating the presence of low muscle mass and low muscle function (strength and performance). It classifies sarcopenia into three stages: presarcopenia, sarcopenia, and severe sarcopenia. Presarcopenia is characterized by low muscle mass, with no impact on physical performance and on strength. Therefore, severe sarcopenia is characterized by very low physical performance and strength [78].

In 2013, EWGSOP and IWGS representatives and international experts from Asia and America gathered to form the International Sarcopenia Initiative (ISI) with the aim of conducting a systematic review of some characteristics of sarcopenia. Specifically, the objectives of the systematic review were (1) to assess the prevalence of sarcopenia using definitions that include both muscle mass and muscle function, as proposed by the EWGSOP and IWGS; and (2) to review nutrition and exercise interventions that used both muscle mass and muscle function as outcomes [77].

Sarcopenia is closely related to musculoskeletal performance, which has potential for rehabilitation and physical conditioning, with consequent restoration of physical capacity. So, physical exercises play an important role in maintaining or slowing down muscle loss. Sedentary lifestyle therefore seems to be a risk factor for sarcopenia in the elderly [79].

Exercise interventions apparently play a role in increasing muscle strength and improving physical performance, but they do not appear to consistently increase muscle mass in frail and sedentary institutionalized elderly individuals. Studies with other populations have not been well established. There are no trials with individuals recruited according to their sarcopenia status. Numerous studies suggest the combination of different types of exercises in a program can improve muscle strength and physical performance [77]. However, it is necessary to standardize exercise protocols for different groups according to their sarcopenia statuses, as proposed by the EWGSOP.

Evaluation of the stages of sarcopenia and application of exercises that are appropriate for each patient's physical and nutritional statuses requires a rigorous protocol that controls for confounding variables. That involves looking into the continuous use of many medications, which can interfere with cell metabolism, and also into diets that are low in proteins and in antioxidant foods. Although nutritional intervention is one of the main approaches to sarcopenia, much of the available evidence comes from short-term protein synthesis studies. According to Cruz-Jentoft, there is a paucity of clinical studies with well-founded evidence about nutritional recommendations for patients with sarcopenia [77].

Sarcopenia, as well as other noncommunicable chronic diseases, is a global concern due to the increase in unhealthy life expectancy. Even in countries with a higher healthy life expectancy, sarcopenia poses a threat to the health of the elderly.

Asia is a rapidly aging region with a huge population, and the impact of sarcopenia in this region is therefore massive. The Asian Working Group for Sarcopenia (AWGS) has encouraged research into sarcopenia in Asia and has gathered the best available evidence from surveys on sarcopenia for establishing a consensus diagnosis. However, few consistent studies exist, especially in southern and southeastern Asia. To make matters worse, the heterogeneity of ethnic groups in the region hinders the standardization and clinical application of studies [80].

Sarcopenia is a geriatric syndrome that predisposes the elderly to diseases and to major postoperative complications. According to Smith, patients subjected to radical cystectomy are at risk of major complications when they develop sarcopenia. Risk stratification may be reinforced by objective measures that assess sarcopenia. Sarcopenia has emerged as a new biomarker for adverse outcomes in many clinical settings associated with cystectomy. It is hypothesized that sarcopenia could be associated with major complications after radical cystectomy for bladder cancer and with death [81].

Although prevalence rates vary across studies, both the incidence and prevalence of sarcopenia increase in aging men and women. Between the ages of 75 and 80 years, the prevalence is higher in men than in women because men have larger muscle loss due to the reduction in growth hormone (GH), insulin-like growth factor (IGF-1), and testosterone levels. Moreover, studies with this age group show that rates vary with ethnicity. Despite the fact that muscle loss is greater in men, sarcopenia in elderly women is also important, since life expectancy and prevalence of functional limitations are higher in the latter. Both men and women at the mean age of 60 years begin to have digestive problems, such as lower uptake of proteins that are necessary for the acquisition of muscle mass from the practice of physical exercises. In this case, nutritional therapy with a professional specialized in preventive geriatrics and in nutrition is recommended. Such treatment is important to avoid the development of sarcopenia and osteoporosis.

It is widely known that the prevalence of sarcopenia is higher among women and that it may be associated with osteoporosis, with the risk of fractures, especially of the hip. Thus, sarcopenia could inflict prolonged suffering on the elderly because of the development of diseases and clinical conditions related to inactivity and to malnutrition.

Chapter 33

LOW BONE MASS AND OSTEOPOROSIS

Low bone mass refers to the loss of bone density during the aging process and at the end of the reproductive period. Sedentary menopausal women usually have quick loss of bone mass, being at a higher risk for osteoporosis when compared with men of the same age. Low bone mass is a physiological condition characterized by a decrease in bone mineral density, mainly of calcium and phosphorus levels, and a precursor to osteoporosis. Low bone mass occurs when bone mass is 10 to 25% lower than normal, according to World Health Organization (WHO) standards. If bone mass is greater than that, it is classified as osteoporosis.

Aside from menopausal women, those with amenorrhea or anorexia nervosa may also develop osteoporosis as a result of low calcium intake, low estrogen levels, or possibly both [19].

Osteoporosis is considered a systemic skeletal disease characterized by low bone mass and deterioration of the bone tissue microarchitecture. It occurs not only because of the loss of bone mass, but also because of deficient formation of the bone structure during remodeling of the bone tissue. In addition, there may be a skeletal disorder characterized by poor bone strength and resistance, predisposing to a larger risk of fractures. It is believed that bone mineral density (BMD) corresponds to approximately 70% of bone strength [82].

Osteoporosis can be classified as primary, which is related to the loss of bone mineral density, and secondary, which may be associated with metabolic and hormonal disorders, such as diabetes and glucocorticoid excess. The risk of fracture, however, depends less on BMD and more on bone quality when compared with primary osteoporosis, but the mechanisms of deterioration of bone quality are not well understood yet, which is in line with some studies that demonstrate incompatibility of BMD with the diagnosis of hip and vertebral fractures [83, 84].

Therefore, bone resistance to fracture is the combination of two main aspects: bone density and quality. Primary osteoporosis can affect both sexes and all age groups, but its prevalence is higher among women than among men. Risks, particularly of vertebral and hip fractures, increase with age.

According to WHO criteria, osteoporosis is diagnosed when BMD is 2.5 standard deviations or more below the average for young adults (T-score equal to or less than -2.5).

In sedentary elderly patients, loss of bone mass can average 1% a year. This rate is considered relatively high and alarming if we consider that a 60-year-old will have lost more than 20% of bone mass by the age of 80 years.

Nowadays, osteoporosis is considered the 21st century's new epidemic and a major public health problem that puts future elderly generations at risk. Accordingly, WHO launched the decade of bone and joint (Bone and Joint Decade, 2000-2010) in 1999. The primary goals were a 25% reduction in the expected increase of osteoporotic fractures, whose number had doubled in the decade before. According to WHO, 40% of women aged over 50 years will have osteoporotic fractures in the future [85].

Studies have shown a prevalence rate of 25% or higher for vertebral fractures in women aged over 50 years. Vertebral fractures are often asymptomatic, and only one-third of them are recognized as clinical symptomatic fractures. In this case, fractures can occur even if BMD is above a T-score of -2.5, due to poor bone quality [84]. However, clinical assessment of "bone quality" is not fully developed yet, and the diagnosis of osteoporosis has relied mainly on BMD.

Currently, dual energy X-ray absorptiometry (DEXA) has been the assay most widely used in clinical studies and assessments for the diagnosis of bone mineral density.

Knowingly, mechanical loading is essential for maintenance of bone mass and of its structural integrity. Consequently, reduced physical activity is a risk factor for osteoporosis in the general population. [86] According to researcher and pediatrician Anne-Lise Carrié Fässler, predisposition to osteoporosis begins in childhood and adolescence. More than 90% of bone content in adulthood is acquired during childhood and adolescence. Therefore, children who perform high-impact exercises, such as jumping rope, running, skipping, etc., on a regular basis, will have a higher bone mineral density in the future than those who practice swimming or who do not practice any physical activity at all, spending most of their time in front of computers and tablets.

Therefore, preventive measures have to be implemented against this disease. Such measures should be implemented during childhood and adolescence and maintained in adulthood, thereby ensuring functional independence and good quality of life during old age.

Chapter 34

Chronic Obstructive Pulmonary Disease (COPD)

Chronic obstructive pulmonary disease (COPD) is defined as a common preventable, and sometimes treatable, chronic inflammatory disease. It is characterized by persistent and usually progressive airflow limitation in the airways and lungs associated with an increased chronic inflammatory response triggered by harmful particles or gases, particularly inhaled cigarette smoke. COPD is currently recognized as a complicated systemic disease with several comorbidities, including lung cancer, atherosclerosis, sarcopenia, osteoporosis, diabetes, anxiety, and depression. Some studies have predicted that COPD may rank third as the leading cause of premature death in the world by 2020 [87].

Management of these comorbidities is clinically important, since they are associated with hospitalization, mortality, and poor quality of life. Osteoporosis is one of the major comorbidities of COPD. Although the pathophysiological relationship between COPD and osteoporosis remains to be established, recent epidemiological studies clearly indicate that osteoporosis is highly prevalent in COPD patients [88].

In a retrospective cohort study of 234 male subjects referred for osteoporosis treatment at a single orthopedic clinic, COPD was found to be the major cause of secondary osteoporosis. In addition, osteoporosis-related fractures may further deteriorate lung function and impair daily activities in COPD patients. Both diseases therefore engender a vicious circle, placing a heavy burden on these patients [89].

The question of whether the risk of fracture associated with COPD is more closely related to loss of bone quality or to BMD critically influences the therapeutic strategy to be adopted.

In a clinical study conducted by Lidwien Gract-Verboon (2012) over a three-year period, patients diagnosed with COPD were observed in order to identify risk factors for osteoporosis. The prevalence of osteoporosis increased from 47 to 61% within three years, with risk of hip and vertebral fractures. In addition, the study showed that vitamin D deficiency could increase the risk of fractures by more than sevenfold [89].

Vertebral fractures in COPD patients with prevalence rates between 24 and 79% were reported in other studies. Curiously enough, other studies described thoracic fractures, which were more frequent in the middle of the thoracic region (T7-T8) and at the thoracolumbar junction (T12-L1) rather than in the lumbar region [89]. However, the prevalence of thoracic fractures is still a matter of controversy and requires further investigation in COPD patients.

In general, approximately two-thirds of vertebral fractures prevalent in COPD are asymptomatic and only a small fraction of fractures are recognized as symptomatic clinical fractures. Thus, morphometric analyses of fractures through a spinal X-ray are extremely important. Various studies report a very high prevalence of vertebral fractures in this population. These rates vary widely depending on personal characteristics, such as age and sex, as well as on the severity of COPD [88].

In vivo evaluation of bone quality is quite limited, interfering with the treatment strategies for these patients. Bone biopsy is the only currently available method for the assessment of bone microarchitecture. It allows for direct evaluation of bone microarchitecture at the tissue level. There is only one report on histomorphometric analysis of bone specimens obtained from biopsies of postmenopausal women with COPD not treated with systemic glucocorticoids. The women assessed in such study had a significant reduction in trabecular bone volume and in connectivity density, decreased cortical width, and increased cortical porosity, in comparison with age-matched postmortem control samples [88].

Rapid weight loss is a striking and visible feature in COPD patients, particularly in advanced stages of the disease. In general, body mass index (BMI) is a determinant factor for BMD and for risk of fracture. A very low BMI may be predictive of osteoporosis and severe sarcopenia, also known as cachexia [91]. Cachexia is the last stage of severe sarcopenia, accompanied by serious diseases such as cancer, congenital cardiomyopathy, and end-stage renal disease.

In addition to these consequences, COPD also results from systemic inflammation, with high levels of cytokines (e.g., TNF-α, IL-1, and IL-6), and higher oxidative stress, caused by constant smoking-related lung injuries.

Both *in vitro* and *in vivo* studies suggest that TNF-α, IL-1, and IL-6 induce the formation of osteoclasts (cells involved in bone matrix resorption and bone remodeling) and that they play a role in the pathogenesis of primary and secondary osteoporosis [89].

Note that bone remodeling in COPD patients is a continuous process, and the balance between resorption and ossification is therefore affected. The balance between resorption (osteoclastogenesis) and new bone formation (osteoblastogenesis) is critical for maintaining bone mass and quality.

Systemic inflammation is a pathophysiological process of COPD characterized by mucosal, submucosal, and glandular tissue infiltration by inflammatory cells in the airways, increasing the amount of mucus and epithelial hyperplasia, leading to airway wall thickening. Chronic inflammation and the imbalance between proteases and their inhibitors, which cause problems in tissue repair, lead to the narrowing, obliteration, and destruction of terminal bronchioles [91].

In addition to the normal process of aging and to the environmental and genetic factors our bodies have to cope with over the years, smoking speeds up the whole process and causes many comorbidities, besides pain, prolonged suffering, and premature death.

Chapter 35

ANXIETY DISORDER

According to WHO, the incidence of anxiety disorder has risen significantly in recent years, showing a 33% increase worldwide.

Anxiety is very common among the elderly and may develop as a primary anxiety disorder or have symptoms that mimic those of other diseases, such as dementia and depression. This disorder usually emerges in early adulthood, after the age of 60 years, and could be triggered by a traumatic event.

Recent studies have suggested anxiety disorder, or psychological disorders in general, have a genetic component; however, the environment plays a major role.

Anxiety is characterized by clearly defined psychosomatic signs and symptoms, which include sweating, feelings of suffocation, palpitations, oscillating blood pressure, paresthesia, constant muscle tension, tremors, nausea, diarrhea, and, in some cases, an unknown physical condition.

Psychological signs and symptoms include fear, apprehension, exaggerated worry, insecurity, and irritability, in addition to changes in cognitive functions.

Chapter 36

TYPES OF ANXIETY DISORDERS

PANIC DISORDER

Frequent panic attacks, consisting of mild episodes with sudden onset, considerable apprehension, extreme fear and terror, usually associated with feelings of imminent death.

AGORAPHOBIA

Anxiety about, or avoidance of, places or situations from which escaping could be difficult or embarrassing, or where relief may not be possible in the event of a panic attack.

OBSESSIVE-COMPULSIVE DISORDER

Obsession that can cause deep anxiety or disturbance and/or compulsion, which serves to dispel anxiety.

Generalized Anxiety Disorder: Specific Phobias

At least six months of anxiety and persistent and excessive apprehension. Clinically significant anxiety caused by exposure to a particular object or feared situation, usually triggering an avoidance behavior.

Social Phobia

Avoidance behavior. Social isolation.

Posttraumatic Stress Disorder

Recall of an extremely traumatic event, accompanied by symptoms of increased alertness and avoidance of trauma-associated stimuli [18]. Studies on anxiety disorder present significant data on its prevalence, which is higher among females and among individuals with comorbidities and psychiatric disorders. Some studies, however, indicate a lower prevalence in elderly individuals aged over 65 years (4.5 to 5.4%). Anxiety treatment seeks to put an end to the patient's suffering and to improve his/her quality of life and functional capacity. The first step consists in identifying the type of anxiety disorder to adjust the treatment accordingly. However, drug treatment should be implemented judiciously to avoid adverse reactions, drug interactions, and comorbidities. Special attention should be paid to aging-related pharmacokinetic and pharmacodynamic changes. Psychotherapy plays a very important role in eliminating suffering, such as accepting and embracing grief, coming to terms with aging, stopping nourishing fantasies, in addition to improving self-esteem, confidence, and interpersonal relationships.

There are important reports in the scientific literature that demonstrate anxiety disorder can be mitigated with the practice of physical exercises targeted at controlling movement and breathing, including Pilates exercises, yoga, and tai chi, among others.

Thus, non-pharmacological treatment, such as psychotherapy and specific physical exercises, may be important alternatives for treating this disorder, ensuring well-being and better quality of life for these patients.

Chapter 37

Depressive Disorder

Depressive disorders last longer and are much more serious, being one of the major causes of suicide, reaping the lives of more than 300,000 Americans every year. This disorder is characterized by feelings of failure to control one's emotional state, with sudden onset, often without any apparent cause and, if left untreated, it may persist for several months [18]. Depression in the elderly has a nonspecific and atypical clinical presentation. Estimations indicate that it will be the second largest disorder in developed countries and the first one in developing countries by 2020. The prevalence in the general population ranges from 3 to 11% and it is twice as high among women [20].

Several are the risk factors that predispose the elderly to depression. The social factor has a strong influence on behavior, and social isolation is the main manifestation of this disorder. Depression is more frequent in the elderly because of several factors that are present in this stage of life, such as grieving, severe and chronic diseases, their children's moving away, and lower purchasing power, among others.

In depressive disorder, there may be loss of recent memory and cognitive impairment. These complaints may subside or even cease with proper treatment.

As with anxiety, the use of psychotherapy to treat depression, combined with regular practice of specific exercises can reverse this condition in the elderly and improve quality of life.

Chapter 38

DEMENTIA

We know that the population has been aging all over the world, including some African countries, where life expectancy is lowest. As a result, there has been some concern about the physical and mental status of future generations of elderly people. Life expectancy has increased, but so has the prevalence of dementia in all regions of the world. Epidemiological studies consistently indicate that the prevalence of dementia increases with age and can double every five years between the ages of 65 and 85 years. Epidemiological studies carried out in Brazil suggest a tendency towards a larger number of cases of dementia in poorly educated individuals, based on population samples from some Brazilian regions. However, in the southern and southeastern states, aging and schooling levels are closer to those observed in industrialized countries.

There are several classifications of dementia. Alzheimer's disease (AD), for example, is prevalent in all continents, when compared with the other types of dementia, such as vascular dementia (VD). AD accounts for approximately 60% of the cases of dementia, whereas VD is observed in more than 20%. The effect of age on these two etiological diagnoses can also be observed by looking at the significant increase in the AD to VD ratio in individuals aged over 100 years. The higher AD to VD ratio in centenarians indicates a greater influence of age on AD than on VD.

Table 2. EURODEM – Prevalence rate

Age	Men	Women
30 – 59	0.16%	0.09%
60 – 64	1.58%	0.47%
65 – 69	2.17%	1.10%
70 – 74	4.61%	3.86%
75 – 79	5.04%	6.67%
80 – 84	12.12%	13.50%
85 – 89	18.45%	22.76%
90 – 94	32.1%	32.25%
95 – 99	31.58%	36.0%

Sex-wise, prevalence has increased among women older than 75 years.

There are also other types of dementia that are considered rare, such as hydrocephalic dementia, prion dementia (Creutzfeldt-Jakob disease), and frontotemporal dementia.

Several studies indicate a higher incidence of AD in women older than 75 years, whereas VD is more frequent in men as a consequence of smoking, as suggested by some studies.

The EURODEM study detected an increased risk of AD in current smokers, especially among men, even when this variable was controlled for family history of dementia, cerebrovascular disease, and stroke [92]. Frontotemporal dementia is a pre-senile form of primary degeneration that affects mainly the anterior prefrontal and temporal regions of the brain. Its clinical picture consists primarily of changes in personality and behavior. [93] It is known that Pilates exercises have a positive impact on the general health of adults and elderly. However, whether this exercise program is effective in improving cognitive functions and memory in individuals with VD and AD remains to be known.

Chapter 39

PILATES METHOD AND AGING

Pilates, in his second book, asserted that longevity could be achieved through active aging, with good quality of life and lucidity. He said that: "The art of Contrology proves that the only real guide to your true age lies not in years or how you think you feel but as you actually are as infallibly indicated by the degree of natural and normal flexibility enjoyed by your spine throughout life."

He was genuinely concerned about eating habits in modern times and he himself consumed and advised the consumption of natural foods: "The man who uses intelligence with respect to his diet, his sleeping habits, and who exercises properly, is beyond any question of doubt taking the very best preventive medicines provided so freely and abundantly by nature. Only by doing this you will be able to achieve longevity with good quality of life and lucidity."

He also believed that someone with an active body and balanced mind could succeed in all cognitive, physical, and intellectual tasks, regardless of age. Therefore, the Pilates method plays a crucial role in the prevention of aging-related diseases, especially those that affect the musculoskeletal and cardiac systems.

On the other hand, a sedentary lifestyle in old age produces some chain reactions, initially with progressive loss of muscle and bone mass, which predisposes to the risk of severe fractures. Moreover, such losses are detrimental to several systems, chiefly to the proprioceptive system, causing loss of balance. Proprioception, which was discussed in the musculoskeletal system, informs the brain what is going on in our body in response to the external environment, allowing us to maintain balance through the interaction of muscle fibers, which work to keep the body on its base of support, to recognize the proper position of this base, and to activate the vestibular system, located in the inner ear.

Thus, loss of balance in the elderly is the main cause of falls and, consequently, of severe fractures. According to some studies, falls make elderly people extremely vulnerable, with severe and irreversible consequences, eventually leading to functional impairment and premature death.

In the USA, an elderly person dies every 30 minutes from fall-related injuries, and over 30% of the falls result in incapacitating conditions, such as hip fracture and head trauma, causing premature death [94].

Chapter 40

BALANCE AND PILATES METHOD

Loss of balance in the elderly is associated with many factors that may increase the risk of falls. Some of these factors are considered to trigger loss of balance. The physiological decline that comes with inactive aging is believed to cause higher vulnerability and inability to react properly in a risky situation. The degenerative process that affects the musculoskeletal system, especially in inactive elderly individuals, is likely to cause loss of balance and postural alteration, such as lack of axial alignment, which hinders the elderly people's ability to perceive their center of gravity. In addition, there are other diseases such as sarcopenia and osteoporosis that also deteriorate the musculoskeletal system.

Other factors could contribute towards falls, such as sugar metabolism disorders, known as Ménière's disease.

According to Bittar, there has been an overconsumption of refined sugar in the past decades, and our bodies have not had enough time to adapt to high sugar intake, leading to hyperinsulinemia with consequent reactive hypoglycemia, in addition to other symptoms, including headache, drowsiness, dizziness, and vertigo with tinnitus. This syndrome can occur at any age, but its prevalence is higher among postmenopausal women [95].

Other very common factors that could lead to falls include inner ear infections (labyrinthitis) and continuous use of inappropriate medications (e.g., benzodiazepines) that may cause dizziness and risk of falls.

It is widely known that falls in elderly individuals translate into poor quality of life with prolonged suffering. That is why preventive geriatrics and gerontology play an important role in encouraging scientific studies that prove the efficiency of exercises in achieving and maintaining balance for functional independence and good quality of life.

Pilates exercises are acclaimed in the scientific community because of their safety and efficiency in providing balance, even to sick or debilitated individuals.

Numerous studies have shown strong evidence of the positive effects of Pilates exercises on the body and mind of patients at high risk of falls. These exercises are also indicated as a way to prevent falls in this population.

Systematic reviews and meta-analyses on the efficacy of Pilates exercises in the prevention and treatment of elderly individuals at risk of falls are unanimous about the positive effects on static and dynamic balance, acquisition of strength, flexibility, and improvement in posture.

It is clearly evident that the Pilates method is very efficient in the achievement and maintenance of static and dynamic balance in elderly individuals and young adults. Besides conventional conditioning exercises, the method also includes proprioceptive exercises in an easy-to-learn and periodized order. Bullo suggests that the exercise protocol should be performed in two weekly sessions with moderate workout [96]. The exercises are often performed on apparatuses devised by Pilates, but some of them are carried out with balls and on mats.

Therefore, all exercises are important for the rehabilitation and physical conditioning of elderly people. Moreover, it should be noted that the practice of these exercises allows elderly people to gain more confidence and feel safer in their daily activities, thus improving their quality of life and functional independence.

Currently, many long-established institutions have included Pilates exercises in their routine for rehabilitation and prevention of falls [97].

A clinical study was conducted in an elderly community in Texas (USA) comparing Pilates exercises with a conventional exercise program for rehabilitation of balance. The Pilates method proved to be more efficient in enhancing balance when compared with conventional physical therapy [98].

The key feature of the Pilates method is the correct application of basic exercises along with the principles of the method. Its aim is to raise students' awareness of their bodies and to exert control over their movements, thereby establishing the connection between body and mind. As pointed out by studies on the incidence of falls among elderly individuals, these exercises improve postural stability, strength, flexibility, and balance, and also enhance quality of life and functional independence.

Chapter 41

CANCER AND PILATES METHOD

Cancer, like other chronic diseases mentioned so far, is a treatable disease if a preventive diagnosis is made. Nowadays, therapies are more effective than a few years ago. With scientific breakthroughs, we know to what extent environmental factors influence the development of this controversial disease. Genetic predisposition exists; however, the gene responsible for the disease depends on stimuli from many environmental factors to be activated or silenced. According to Frank W. Booth et al., changes in gene expression induced by a sedentary lifestyle contribute to the development of comorbidities and mortality. Therefore, physical exercises shape physiological responses, defined by the induction of physical exercises [39].

In recent years, more variables have emerged that can alter organic homeostasis and contribute to the development of the disease, such as increase of emotional stress, consumption of industrialized foods, smoking, and close contact with chemical agents and pollutants.

Today, the scientific community seeks to add a rehabilitation treatment to cancer therapy in order to reduce the aggressive symptoms triggered by conventional treatment. Currently, there has been a great deal of interest in investigating the effects of Pilates training on people subjected to cancer treatment, especially in the case of breast cancer.

Many systematic reviews and meta-analyses have shown the positive effects of Pilates exercises on breast cancer patients. These studies have reported significant improvements in the physical and psychological statuses as well as in the quality of life of these patients (improvement in mood and body image). [99] Generally, these patients who experience a great deal of emotional stress due to the effects of anticancer treatment become more physically and emotionally vulnerable. In addition to surgical trauma and exhausting chemotherapy and radiation therapy, the patient may develop various disorders, especially anxiety disorder, depression, and sleep disorders.

After chemotherapy or radiation therapy, physical toxicity persists for a long time. The patient's quality of life is impaired, including unpleasant symptoms such as lymphedema (swelling in one or more extremities caused by surgery and radiation therapy), neuropathy (depending on the type of chemotherapy), fatigue, arthralgia (joint pain), and biomechanical dysfunctions. [100] Lymphedema is the accumulation of fluids in soft tissues resulting from impaired flow of the lymphatic system. The lymphatic system is not able to effectively drain the lymphatic fluids from a given region of the body due to changes in lymphatic structure or function. This may occur after the treatment of breast cancer, but it can also be observed in other types of cancer.

Pilates exercises improve the capacity of the muscular, respiratory, and cardiovascular systems, controlling physical and mental stress, thus facilitating lymphatic drainage. Moreover, specificity of movements, such as arm and leg circle exercises, can stimulate recovery in lymph nodes.

In the clinical study by Sener et al., Pilates exercises proved to be effective in patients with lymphedema, reducing fluid accumulation and, consequently, improving the quality of life. [101]

Biomechanical dysfunctions in breast cancer patients initially occur in the upper limbs, consequently affecting the whole musculoskeletal system and compromising strength, flexibility, and motor coordination. Radiation therapy and cancer surgery may induce progressive fibrosis and scarring that contribute to denervation of the motor endplate [100].

Thus, effective strategies are needed for the treatment and recovery of physiological functions in these patients. These strategies should contribute to eliminating intoxication caused by chemotherapy and radiation therapy, and to treating emotional disorders associated with the disease. Recent studies have shown that active people are more likely to recover than sedentary individuals. Therefore, research studies suggest endurance exercises for fighting fatigue, a very common consequence of conventional breast cancer treatment.

Pilates exercises can aid in eliminating the toxic effects of radiation therapy and chemotherapy, in addition to facilitating the restoration of shoulder mobility, increasing muscle strength, and relieving the pain associated with breast surgery, thus improving the daily skills and quality of life in these patients. At the time when Pilates lived, there were few reports on cancer, and there was not any treatment other than surgery. In the case of breast cancer, radical mastectomy was the standard procedure.

Eve Gentry had breast cancer at that time and underwent mastectomy. For a dancer, that meant stepping away from one's career for several years. However, Pilates, based on his empirical research, believed his method could be effective in restoring shoulder mobility and relieving the pain associated with mastectomy.

Chapter 42

EVE GENTRY'S STORY

In 1955, Eve Gentry, a ballet dancer and choreographer who worked as a Pilates assistant, was diagnosed with breast cancer. At the time, mastectomy was the only available intervention, and many patients were unable to work after undergoing such procedure. However, Eve trusted in Pilates' work and talent. A few days after the surgery, Eve asked Pilates whether her arm movements could ever be restored. And he simply replied, "Do not worry, we will fix them."

In New York, one year after her surgery, Eve could dance again, and she performed a number where her arms moved normally. She believed Pilates was largely responsible for her total recovery.

In 1994, Eve died shortly before turning 85. She had been teaching until the last years of her life, when her health started to collapse. Eve was a brilliant and innovative teacher, greatly admired by her followers. Her philosophy and mastery of movements were a major contribution to the teaching of the Pilates method [102].

At that time, she was held up as an example for having overcome an incurable disease, which often had serious physical and psychological sequelae. In addition to regaining joint mobility and muscle strength with the exercises carefully planned and periodized by Pilates, she also learned how to overcome physical pain and come to terms with her mutilated body.

Today, even with the advent of scientific advancements, 50 to 80% of cancer patients suffer from pain of varying intensity, caused either by the disease itself or by treatment.

Chapter 43

Chronic Pain and Pilates Method

We are currently living in a time when research has developed very quickly and scientific breakthroughs have abounded; nevertheless, many people still suffer from chronic pain and more and more individuals go through psychological pain.

Chronic pain can have some implications for quality of life. It is usually accompanied by emotional stress, possibly resulting in depressive disorders, anxiety, fatigue, poor concentration, and social isolation.

The chapter on the musculoskeletal system dealt with the importance of acute pain, which acts like an alarm, warning us about some aggressive event inflicted on the body. This type of pain is temporary and treatable. However, chronic pain is multifactorial. If left untreated, symptoms may aggravate. Treatment by a multidisciplinary team is then advisable, depending on the type of pain and on the severity of symptoms.

Scientific studies on Pilates exercise interventions in patients with chronic pain, especially low back pain, are en vogue at present. Several volunteers report total relief of low back pain and improvement of joint mobility after Pilates exercises when compared with conventional physical therapy [103]. Women who have reached menopause usually say: "At this stage, it is normal to feel pain all over the body." In most cases, the cause of pain is multifactorial. However, in addition to the normal aging process, physical inactivity is the main cause of muscle and joint pain, and it also increases the risk of developing osteoporosis and other complications over time. Chronic low back pain is a musculoskeletal disorder with a high prevalence in many developed countries. It is estimated that more than 80% of people living in these countries suffer or have already suffered from low back pain.

The etiology of this pathology is still a great hindrance to its treatment and diagnosis, since it is considered a complex health problem that is heterogeneous and multifactorial. It usually occurs concomitantly with degenerative, mechanical, and postural disorders, which are regarded as triggers of chronic low back pain, either separately or in combination with another spinal segment [104]. According to Hayflick (1996), musculoskeletal disorders are among the most prevalent and symptomatic problems at this stage of life.[105]. Nowadays, the Pilates method is widely used to achieve therapeutic goals and it is often recommended by many health professionals.

The benefits of the Pilates method are supported by scientific evidence, which shows its positive effects on health, quality of life, and physical performance. Although the method lacks standardization of some parameters, such as intervention time, exercise levels, and classification of mat exercises or those performed on apparatuses, many studies have a consensus agreement that Pilates exercises are better than conventional rehabilitation exercises as they allow for faster and long-lasting results. Da Luz et al. compared basic Pilates exercises performed on apparatuses and on mats. They found out those exercises performed on apparatuses were better than mat exercises, demonstrating positive effects on the relief of nonspecific low back pain and on the elimination of kinesiophobia [106].

In postmenopausal women with symptoms of chronic low back pain, Pilates exercises seem to have additional benefits when compared with conventional physical therapy, which consists of joint mobilization and electrotherapy. Alleviation of pain and disability with Pilates exercises lasts longer and can be observed after a one-year follow-up [107].

Chapter 44

DEGENERATIVE DISEASES AND PILATES METHOD

The major neurodegenerative disorders include Alzheimer's disease, Parkinson's disease, and trinucleotide repeat disorders (Huntington's and spinocerebellar ataxias). These disorders affect nearly 5 million people in the United States and more than 25 million people worldwide.

Most of these diseases emerge at midlife or later, and aging may actually contribute to susceptibility [38]. Late-onset neurodegenerative diseases are conceptually grouped into two categories: sporadic (of unknown etiology) and hereditary. Alzheimer's and Parkinson's diseases are predominantly sporadic; hereditary forms affect only a small number of patients [38].

Chapter 45

PARKINSON'S DISEASE

Parkinson's disease is a chronic and progressive neurological disease, which affects the movements of the body. It occurs when dopamine-producing nerve cells die or are impaired. Dopamine is a chemical messenger that transmits signals from the *substantia nigra* to another part of the brain called *corpus striatum*, controlling coordinated movement. When these cells die, the other movement control areas in the brain become dysregulated.

The etiology of Parkinson's disease is uncertain in most patients, who are considered to suffer from "sporadic" Parkinson's disease. It is believed, however, that the disorder results from a combination of genetic and environmental factors. Exposure to environmental toxins, such as pesticides, underlies the association of Parkinson's disease with rural life and with the consumption of well water [38]. Many of these components are mitochondrial toxins that can damage dopaminergic cells by interfering with their energy metabolism. Monogenic mutations (dominant gene between families) are also responsible for activating the disease-related gene [38]. Parkinson's disease develops gradually, starting at times with a slightly remarkable tremor on one hand. Over time, stiffness affects the whole body, causes postural imbalance, slows down movements, and alters speech.

According to the National Parkinson Foundation (Parkinson.org), Parkinson's disease is the second most common neurodegenerative disease, outranked by Alzheimer's disease. It affects men and women equally. It does not have any predilection for social class, ethnic group, economic status, or geographical region. In the United States, it is estimated that 60,000 new cases are diagnosed each year, adding to 1.5 million Americans currently living with Parkinson's disease. Although this condition usually develops after the age of 65 years, 15% of diagnosed individuals are younger than 50 years [109].

Each person presents with a unique set of symptoms, which worsen with time. Drug treatment is aimed at reducing specific symptoms and often consists of combination therapy. The combination of drugs depends on the patient's tolerance to them. Parkinson's disease is often treated with dopaminergic medications, which have a number of side effects, such as nausea, low blood pressure, dyskinesia (twitching), and hallucinations. Many patients need more medication over time, which tends to exacerbate the side effects [108].

Over the past 50 years, surgery has been used to relieve symptoms such as incapacitating tremors and dyskinesia. The latest surgical approach is known as deep brain stimulation (DBS), a technique developed in the 1990s and approved by the FDA in 1997. DBS involves the insertion of electrodes into a target area of the brain, determined by the patient's symptoms, and the implantation of a device under the collarbone. The device provides direct current and acts upon motor function. DBS does not help improve balance or freezing of gait, and it is only minimally effective in improving speech and posture. However, in addition to all these alternatives for temporary symptom relief, a lot of research is being done on the effects of physical exercise on the treatment of Parkinson's disease.

Today, recent neuroplasticity studies have shown the importance of stimulation through exercises. Neuroscientist Anthony Hannan, head of the Neural Plasticity Laboratory at the Florey Institute of Neuroscience and Mental Health, along with T.Y.C Pang and other researchers, conducted a series of experiments with mice, changing our understanding of the role of environment and exercise in altering the course of catastrophic genetic neurodegenerative disorders [109]. While it is openly acknowledged that Parkinson's disease is incurable, daily exercises of a very specific type are believed to reverse the worst symptoms of the disease or halting its progression in certain cases. Current applications that contain songs that guide the walking pace of patients with Parkinson's disease are available. These applications can be downloaded by patients to their own cell phones. At the onset of the walking training, patients should be guided and supervised by a professional. This guidance occurs according to the stage of the disease in which the training was initiated. This way, patients can gain autonomy over time.

At present, studies on Pilates exercise intervention in patients with Parkinson's disease are lacking. In June 2011, Brent Anderson, president and CEO of Polestar Pilates Center in Miami (FL), presented a study with a small group of patients with Parkinson's disease at the 6th World Congress of the International Society of Physical & Rehabilitation Medicine in San Juan (Puerto Rico). His findings were encouraging, as all volunteers reported a reduction of symptoms and improvement in quality of life. Just like Brent Anderson, other professionals conducted interesting studies with positive results. Some of these studies are not official, though.

Interesting studies that evaluated balance in fall-prone patients have also been carried out. In addition to improved balance, patients enhanced joint mobility and developed greater confidence while performing their daily activities. Therefore, Pilates exercises may be regarded as an excellent method for helping alleviate some of the motor symptoms of Parkinson's disease, such as stiffness, weakness, slow movements, impaired pelvic floor control, loss of balance, and poor posture. Despite the paucity of evidence-based studies on the effectiveness of Pilates exercises in this population, the case studies presented so far suggest improvements in motor and non-motor symptoms commonly observed in Parkinson's disease. Depression, anxiety, cognitive impairment, and sleep disorders are non-motor signs and symptoms with very poor response to dopamine replacement therapy. These signs appear as the disease progresses, impairing quality of life. Besides improving motor symptoms, Pilates exercises can restore patients' confidence and autonomy when they apply the principles of the method.

Controlled clinical trials with significant samples are needed to prove the efficacy of Pilates exercises in delaying the progression of the symptoms and enhancing the quality of life of patients with Parkinson's disease. Recall that Pilates, in his teachings, always stressed the importance of focusing on the movements during exercise. He said: "Correctly executed and mastered to the point of subconscious reaction, these exercises will reflect grace and balance in your routine activities. Contrology exercises build a sturdy body and sound mind fitted to perform every daily task with ease and perfection as well as to provide tremendous reserve energy for sports, recreation, emergencies. [9]"

Additional studies suggest the Pilates method can relieve mental stress, increase oxygen supply to the brain, and improve brain function. However, direct evidence (e.g., electroencephalographic findings) of positive effects of the method on brain activity is lacking. Zhijie Bian et al. assessed the effect of Pilates exercises on the brain function of a group of young female volunteers (five case studies). They found that the alpha rhythm changes during Pilates training in different regions of the brain. The whole brain was analyzed, primarily by means of power spectral density and of the global synchronization index (GSI). The neural network was more active, whereas synchronization strength decreased in the frontal and temporal regions as a result of Pilates training [25]. These findings support the evidence that Pilates exercises are quite efficient in improving brain function or intelligence. This suggests that Pilates training is very useful in the treatment of neurodegenerative diseases and rehabilitation of cognitive functions [25].

Chapter 46

MULTIPLE SCLEROSIS

Multiple sclerosis is primarily an inflammatory disease of the brain and of the spinal cord, in which focal lymphocytic infiltration leads to myelin and axonal damage. In some cases, this disease can also affect the optic nerve. Initially, inflammation is transient and remyelination, albeit present, is short-lived [111]. The onset of the disease is characterized by episodes of neurological dysfunction that usually resolve themselves. Over time, pathological changes cause generalized microglial activation associated with extensive and chronic brain degeneration, with progressive development of a large variety of deficiencies [110]. Multiple sclerosis affects more than 2.5 million people worldwide, especially those aged between 20 and 40 years, and its incidence is twice as high in women [111]. The diagnostic criteria for multiple sclerosis were originally formulated by McDonald et al. (2001) and revised by Polman et al. (2005, 2011). All of these criteria rely on conventional magnetic resonance imaging.

Usually, 85% of patients with multiple sclerosis experience its first symptom, the so-called clinically isolated syndrome, which reappears after having been apparently cured. Two-thirds of these patients will develop a secondary progressive form, while the other third will follow a benign course [112]. The remainder of the patients with multiple sclerosis (15%)

will directly develop a primary progressive form. Owing to the different forms of disease progression, different symptoms may be present, such as fatigue, weakness, postural instability, and cognitive disorders. Previous studies with aerobic and endurance exercises showed significant improvements in muscle strength, exercise tolerance, and mobility in patients with multiple sclerosis [113].

In the scientific literature, there has been strong evidence of the efficacy of Pilates exercises applied to vulnerable individuals. Thus, the Pilates method could contribute to suppressing the symptoms that may arise with the progression of the disease.

According to Tomruk et al., Pilates exercises proved to be effective in controlling posture and reducing fatigue in multiple sclerosis patients [114].

In another study, Pilates exercises were applied to wheelchair-bound multiple sclerosis patients. The study revealed significant improvements in adapted functional performance tests, in posture, in pain relief, and in daily living skill activities. The qualitative component of this study also confirmed that Pilates lessons are beneficial and fun for wheelchair-bound multiple sclerosis patients. Therefore, the benefits assessed and perceived by participants may increase the likelihood of long-term adherence to the exercise programs [115].

Degenerative diseases affect millions of people around the world, and most of these diseases are sporadic and of unknown etiology. Several studies are then carried out in an attempt to find the cure for these diseases.

While no compelling evidence of cure of these diseases is obtained, preventive measures should be taken to slow down the progression of these diseases or minimize their distressing symptoms. Currently, many health professionals recognize the importance of adopting preventive strategies, such as nutritional care and regular physical exercise, as a way to reduce the adverse effects of conventional treatments, which are often aggressive and debilitating.

Therefore, analyzing these possible aging-related events reinforces the idea that lifestyle change is a way to guarantee good-quality aging in this new era with extended lifespan.

Chapter 47

QUALITY OF LIFE

Quality of life can be assessed through a method used to measure a person's living conditions or a set of conditions that contribute to the well-being of individuals in society. It involves physical, spiritual, psychological, and emotional well-being, in addition to social relationships. Preventive geriatrics plays an important role in maintaining quality of life in all stages of life. It structurally falls into the pattern followed by preventive pediatrics [20].

Preventive geriatrics can be approached in three different ways. Primary preventive geriatrics includes all actions aimed at reducing or delaying the emergence of age-related chronic degenerative disorders and morbidities. Secondary preventive geriatrics relies on the diagnosis and early treatment of chronic degenerative disorders and morbidities. And, finally, tertiary preventive geriatrics is aimed at providing some guidance to individuals who already suffer from age-related diseases, preventing their relapse [42].

Quality of life has taken on added importance in many respects in recent years, particularly with regard to its assessment or measurement, either individually or collectively.

Both therapeutic and technological advancements have increased the survival of patients, especially of those with chronic diseases.

International organizations have become increasingly interested in having an instrument to evaluate and measure quality of life and that has prompted the World Health Organization (WHO) to devise an instrument for this purpose, which could not only assess the improvement in the survival rates of various diseases, but also the recent rise in the aging population. [116]

Currently, researchers from several countries have been using the WHOQOL-bref, an instrument that evaluates the quality of life of the population being studied. The WHOQOL assesses individuals' perceptions of their status in life in the cultural and value system contexts relative to their goals, expectations, standards, and concerns. It was developed in collaboration with several culturally diverse centers over a four-year period. Despite the fact that this instrument has been developed relatively recently, there has been a great interest in its use in scientific studies. The expansion in the publication of scientific papers helps disseminate and give visibility to the instrument, demonstrating its diverse possibilities of use from an international and cross-cultural perspective. In addition, the WHOQOL-bref can be used in clinical practice as a way to improve the doctor-patient relationship, as an instrument for evaluation and comparison of responses to different treatments, in addition to being useful in public health services. It is a short and easy-to-apply instrument that can be used both in populations with some type of disease and in healthy populations.

These instruments can generate new knowledge, raise questions, and contribute to making decisions that actually improve people's quality of life.

In recent years, there has been great interest in investigating specific exercise programs that deal with the connection between body and mind, as are the cases of the Pilates method and Mindfulness meditation. As these methods seek to integrate body and mind, the outcomes of these practices are positive for all the quality of life parameters analyzed.

A study with university students analyzed high levels of stress, quality of sleep, anxiety, and depression. While numerous Mindfulness-based clinical interventions can effectively reduce stress and other disorders, in this study, some reticent students sought clinical treatment through psychoanalysis. However, this study provides us with encouraging preliminary data suggesting the introduction of exercises with broad and coordinated movements that can arouse the interest of participants and thus effectively increase mindfulness. The development of mindfulness is associated with significant improvements in mood and stress which, in turn, provides better quality of sleep [118]. Many studies indicate that Pilates exercises seem to be an effective physical fitness program for the improvement of quality of life. In a study conducted by Kuçuk with adult women aged 20 to 45 years, significant and positive changes were observed after Pilates exercise interventions. The main changes included satisfaction with one's life, perception of acceptance by other people, perception of physical appearance, and perception of group functionality [119].

In a study with postmenopausal women diagnosed with osteoporosis, the outcomes obtained with the intervention were very encouraging as well. Most participants reported a significant decrease in back pain after the exercise intervention and an increase in functional capacity and, consequently, some improvement in quality of life. [120]

The same result was also found by Natour et al., who evaluated patients with nonspecific chronic low back pain [121]. As with these studies, many other studies on Pilates exercises, carried out with elderly and young adults, describe a significant change in quality of life and well-being.

This way, quality of life is the most important issue, not only for the elderly, but also for all people, at all ages. We should recall, however, that today's young people will be tomorrow's elderly, who will represent everything that was invested in their past.

According to Campos, well-being is a process rather than an objective, which implies a choice and a way of life. This means integrating body, mind, and spirit. It represents acceptance of oneself. This suggests that what one believes and feels affects one's health [122].

For Roh, well-being is classified into five dimensions: (A) physical well-being, which can be defined as the ability to perform daily tasks through physical activity and proper nutrition; (B) social well-being, which is the ability to build healthy and supportive relationships and to establish a strong connection with other people; (C) spiritual well-being, which can be characterized as guidance about the meaning or value in life; (D) intellectual well-being, which may be the ability to learn, to acquire knowledge, and to develop skills, applying them in daily tasks; and (E) emotional well-being, which can be defined as the ability to deal with emotions and express them properly and comfortably [123]. Within this context, we cannot talk about quality of life without referring first to physical and psychological well-being, since both affect other dimensions of well-being. Relieving these often chronic ailments requires recognition of the need to change behaviors as well as cultural and social patterns and, especially, the belief that the healing power is within us. Only by doing that can we reach other dimensions of well-being in order to acquire a healthy lifestyle with good quality of life.

The Pilates method allows for physical and behavioral changes. It means living wisely with joy and satisfaction, giving the body and mind freedom to gain autonomy.

FINAL REMARKS

Living longer and being mindful of how we are living has become a concern all over the world. Inactivity and the prolonged use of continuous medications incur large expenses for the elderly and for the government and directly affect the quality of life of the elderly, who often have to rely on their families and caregivers for their daily activities. However, governmental organizations in several countries have adopted preventive measures aimed at rationalizing medication use, thus avoiding the practice of polypharmacy and its consequences on the health of the elderly population. These are important measures that can urge the elderly to change their behavior and have a more active and healthy lifestyle. The Pilates method differs from many other methods that only provide physical conditioning and rehabilitation. It is more than a simple exercise performed in an automated fashion. As previously demonstrated, the exercises created by Pilates follow an educational order for the movements, with the application of methodological principles that help integrate body and mind. Achieving such goal may be the hardest task because it takes time and requires determination to stick to it. Several practitioners of the Pilates method have stories and encouraging statements about the changes in posture and quality of life attained after the exercise programs.

Therefore, in order to have a healthy and active aging process, people should be cognizant and mindful of their healthcare needs, as this will help them walk the thin line between health and disease. Both discipline and knowledge of basic healthcare are needed, in addition to the guidance of professionals specialized in the prevention of diseases associated with aging and with sedentary lifestyle. Thinking about aging involves considering special care in all stages of life. Knowing how to grow old wisely is to appeal to our intrinsic nature with respect and dignity in every step of the way.

REFERENCES

[1] Roh SY. An exploration of implications for the development of Pilates instructor system through identification of instructor's difficulties. *Journal of Exercise Rehabilitation.* 2016; 12(4):355-362.

[2] Latey P. The Pilates Method History and Philosophy. *Journal of Bodywork and Movement Therapies.* 2001;5(4):275-282.

[3] Camarão T. *Pilates in Brazil.* Elsevier, 2004.

[4] Pinto J. Effectiveness of conventional physical therapy and Pilates method in functionality, respiratory muscle strength and ability to exercise in hospitalized chronic renal patients: study protocol of randomized controlled trial. *Journal of Bodywork and Movement Therapies.* 2015;19:604-615.

[5] Pedriali FR. Is Pilates as effective as conventional pelvic floor muscle exercise in the conservative treatment of post-prostatectomy urinary incontinence? A randomised controlled trial. *Neurology and Urodynamic.* 2016;35:615-621.

[6] *Life Magazine.* August 11, 1947.

[7] Friedman P, Eisen G. *The Pilates Method of physical and mental conditioning - Viking studio,* 2005.

[8] Pilates JH. *Your Health.* Copyright 1998-2008 Presentation Dynamics Inc.

[9] Pilates JH, Miller WJ. *Return to life through Contrology.* Originally Published in 1945.

[10] Campos R. Effect of Pilates method on Physical conditioning of health subjects: a systematic review and meta-analysis. *The Journal of Sports Medicine and Physical Fitness.* 2016;56(7-8):864-873.

[11] Wells C, Kolt G, Bialocerkowski A. A Defining Pilates exercise: a systematic review. *Complementary Therapies in Medicine.* 2012;20:253-262.

[12] Melo M, Gomes L, Silva Y, Bonezi A, Loss J. Assessment of resistance torque and resultant muscular force during Pilates hip extension exercise and its implications to prescription and progression. *Ver. Bras. Fisioter.* 2011;15(1):23-30.

[13] Siler B. Siler B. *The Pilates Body: The Ultimate At-Home Guide to Strengthening, Lengthening and Toning Your Body - Without Machines.* 2000.

[14] Junges S, Gottlieb MGV, Baptista RR, Quadros CB, Resende TL, Gomes I. Effectiveness of Pilates method for the posture and flexibility of women with hyperkyphosis. *Rev. Bras e Mov.* 2012; 20(1):21:33.

[15] Myers TW. *Anatomy Trains.* Churchill Livingstone-Elsevier, 2009.

[16] Massey P. *The Anatomy of Pilates.* Berkeley-Lótus Publishing, 2009.

[17] McArdle, Willian D. *Exercise Physiology: Nutrition, Energy, and Human Performance, s*eventh edition, 2010.

[18] Bear, Mark F. *Neuroscience: exploring the brain,* 2007.

[19] Kenney WL, Wilmore JH, Costill DL. *Physiology of Sport and Exercise,* 2012.

[20] Moriguchi Y. *Preventive geriatric and gerontology – new concepts.* EIPUCRS, 2014.

[21] *American College of Sports Medicine,* 2010.

[22] Barbosa AW, Guedes CA, Bonifácio DN, Silva A, Martin F, Barbosa MC. The Pilates breathing technique increases the electromyographic amplitude level of deep abdominal muscle in untrained people. *Journal of Bodywork - Mov. Terap.* 2015;19:57-61.

[23] Tonico-fernandez M, Martin MJ, Sânchez-Caravaca MA, Fernandez-Pérez A, Ramirez-Rodrigo J, Villaverde-Gutiérez C. The Pilates method and cardiorespiratory adaptation to training. *Research in Sports Medicine*, 2016 - http://www.tandfonline.com/loi/gspm20.

[24] Purves D. *Neuroscience.* Sinauer Associates, Inc., 2001.

[25] Bian Z, Sun H, Lu C, Li Yao, Chen S, Li X. *Effect of Pilates training on Alpha Rhythm.* Hindawi. 2013 – http://dx doi org/10.1155/2013/295986.

[26] *Pilates style.* May/June, 2008.

[27] *Life Magazine*, March 8, Arabella Churchill, 1954.

[28] World Health Organization, 2000.

[29] Junges S, Jacondino CB, Gottlieb MGV. Effect of Pilates exercises in risk factor for cardiometabolic diseases: a systematic review. *Scientia Medica.* 2015; 25(1).

[30] Rupérez AI, Gil A, Aquilera CM. Genetics of Oxidative Stress in Obesity. *International Journal of Molecular Sciences.* 2014;15(2): 3118-3144.

[31] Banerjee M, Vats P. Reactive metabolites and antioxidant gene polymorphisms in type 2 diabetes mellitus. *Indian J Hum Genet.* 2014; 20(1):10-19.

[32] Galasseti P. Inflammation and oxidative stress in obesity, metabolic syndrome and diabetes. *Exp. Diabetes Res.* 2012.

[33] Albert K, Zimmet P, Shaw J. Metabolic syndrome – a new worldwide definition. A consensus statement from the International Diabetes Federation. *Diabetes Med.* 2006;23(5):469-480.

[34] Gottlieb MGV, da Cruz IBM, Bodanese LC. Origin of the metabolic syndrome: genetic evolutionary and nutritional aspects. *Scientia Medica,* 2008;18(1): 31-38.

[35] Junges S, Molina RD, Jacondino CB, Da Poian ML, Tastsch E, Moresco RN, Gottlieb MGV. Effectiveness of Pilates and *Camellia sinensis* supplementation on cardiometabolic risk factor and redox markers in postmenopausal women: A placebo-controlled, randomized trial. *Journal of Aging Research & Clinical Practice.* 2017; 6:80-87.

[36] Junges S, Jacondino CB, Gottlieb MGV. Effect of Pilates exercises in risk factor for cardiometabolic diseases: a systematic review. *Scientia Medica.* 2015;25(1).

[37] Junges S. *Pilates Method: Passion and Science.* AGE/Criterio, 2014.

[38] Kendel ER. *Neuroscience,* 2014.

[39] Booth FW, Chakravarthy MV, Spangemburg EE. *Exercise and gene expression: physiological regulation of human genome through physical activity.* 2002; 543:399-411.

[40] Holliday R. Understanding ageing. *The Royal Society.* 1997;352-363.

[41] Kirkwood TB & Austad SN. Why do we age? *Nature.* 2000;408:233-237.

[42] Moriguchi Y. *Geriatry and gerontology prevention: New concepts,* 2013.

[43] Troen BR. The Biology of Aging. *The Mount Sinai Journal of Medicine.* 2003;70:3-22.

[44] Gottlieb MGV, Carvalho D, Schneider RH, da Cruz IBM. *Genetics aspects of aging and related diseases: a complex network of interactions between genes and environment.* 2007;10(3):273-283.

[45] Kaput J, Rodriguez RL. *Nutritional genomics: The next frontier in the postgenomic error.* 2004; 16(2):166-177.

[46] Barbosa EB, Vidotto A, Polachini GM, Henrique T, Marqui ABT, Tajara EH. *Proteomics: methodologies and applications to the study of human diseases.* 2012; 58:366-375.

[47] Gray MD, Shen JC, Kamath-Loeb AS, Blank A, Sopher BL, Martim GM, Oshima J, Lawrence A. The Werner Syndrome protein is a DNA helicase. *Nature.* 1997; 17:100-103.

[48] Kim HK, Lee JY, Bae HJ. Hutchinson-Giltard Progeria syndrome with G608 LMNA mutation. *J Korean Med Sci.* 2011; 26(12): 1642-1645.

[49] Savela S, Saijanmaa O, Strandberg TE, Koistinen P, Strandberg AY, Tilvis RS, Pikala KH, Miettinen TA, Fyhrquist F. Physical activity in midlife and telomere length measured in old age. *Experimental Gerontology* - Elsevier. 2013;48 (1): 81-84.

[50] Ho SC, Wu S, Chan SG, Show A. Menopausal transition and changes of body composition: a prospective study in Chinese premenopausal women. *International Journal of Obesity.* 2010; 34: 1265-1274.

[51] Marques F, Markus MA, Morris BJ. The molecular basis of longevity, and clinical implications. *Maturitas.* 2010; 65(2): 87-91.

[52] Kappeler L, Epelbaum J. Biological aspects of longevity and ageing. *Ver. Epidemol.* Sante Publique. 2005;53(3): 235-241.

[53] Deisseroth K, Feng G, Majewska AK, Miesenböck G, Ting A, Schnitzer MJ. Next-generation Optical Technologies for Illuminating Genetically Targeted Brain. *Journal of Neuroscience.* 2006; 26(41): 10380-10386.

[54] World Health Organization, 2015.

[55] Gilman CJ; Rhodes, T; et al. The metabolic syndrome and risk of major coronary events in the Scandinavian Simvastatin Survival Study (4S) and the Air Force/Texas Coronary Atherosclerosis Prevention Study (AFCAPS/TexCAPS). *Am J Cardiol.* 2004; 93: 136–141.

[56] Fontana, L; Klein, S. Aging, adiposity, and calorie restriction. *JAMA.* 2007; 297 (9): 986-994.

[57] Gottlib, MGV; et al. *Oxidative stress as an emerging cardiometabolic risk factor.* Scientia Medica (PUCRS Printed -, 2010.

[58] Poljsak, B; Milisav, I. *Aging, oxidative stress and antioxidants, oxidative stress and chronic degenerative diseases.* 2013.

[59] Khan SI, Aumsuwan P, Khan IA, Walker LA, Dasmahapatra AK. Epigenetic events associated with breast cancer and their prevention by dietary components targeting the epigenome. *Chem Res Toxicol.* 2012 Jan 13;25(1):61-73. doi: 10.1021/tx200378c. Epub 2011 Oct 28. Review.

[60] Otani H. Oxidative Stress as Pathogenesis of Cardiovascular Risk Associated with Metabolic Syndrome. *Antioxid Redox Signal.* 2011; 15 (7): 1911-1926.

[61] Rahal A, et al. *Oxidative Stress, Prooxidants, and Antioxidants: The Interplay.* BioMed Research International. 2014.

[62] Yavari A, et al. Exercise-Induced Oxidative Stress and Dietary Antioxidants. *Asian J Sports Med.* 2015; 6 (1): 248-298.

[63] Banerjee M, Vats P. Reactive metabolites and antioxidant gene polymorphisms in Type 2 diabetes mellitus. *Indian J Hum Genet.* 2014; 20 (1): 10-19.

[64] Sousa M, Brás Silva C, Moreira A. O papel da leptina na regulação da homeostasia energética. *Acta Med Port.* 2009; 22: 291-298.

[65] Pandey K, Rizvi S. Resveratrol May Protect Plasma proteins from Oxidation under Conditions of Oxidative Stress *in Vitro*. *J. Braz. Chem. Soc.* 2010; 21 (5): 909-913.

[66] Codoñer-Franch P, et al. Elevated advanced Oxidation protein products (AOPPs) indicate metabolic risk in severely obese children. *Nutrition, Metabolism & Cardiovascular Diseases.* 2012; 22: 237-243.

[67] Benzie IF, Strain JJ. The ferric reducing ability of plasma (FRAP) as a measure of "antioxidant power": the FRAP assay. *Anal Biochem.* 1996; 239 (1): 70-76.

[68] Iris F, et al. Ferric reducing/antioxidant power assay: Direct measure of total antioxidant activity of biological fluids and modified version for simultaneous measurement of total antioxidant power and ascorbic acid concentration. *Circulation: Journal of the American Heart Association.* 2004; 109 (17): 2116-2122.

[69] Morales-González J. Oxidative Stress and Chronic Degenerative Diseases. *A Role for Antioxidants.* Intech: Edition 1. ISBN: 978-953-51-1123-8, 2014.

[70] Otsuka R, et al. Relationship between number of metabolic syndrome components and dietary factors in middle-aged and elderly Japanese subjects. *Hypertens Res.* 2010; 33 (6): 548-554.

[71] Pimentel CVM, Francki VM, Gollücke APB. *Functional foods: introduction to the main bioactive substances in foods.* São Paulo: Livraria Varela, 2005.

[72] Crozier A, Clifford MN, Astrihara H. *Plant secondary Metabolites.* Blackwell Publishing, 2006.

[73] Vieira Senger AE, Schwanke CHA, Gottlieb MGV. Green tea (*Camellia sinensis*) and its functional properties in chronic diseases. *Scientia Medica* (Porto Alegre). 2010; 20 (4): 292-300.

[74] Cabrera M, et al. Metabolic syndrome, abdominal obesity, and cardiovascular risk in elderly women. *Int J Cardiol.* 2007; 114: 224-229.

[75] Basu A, Lucas E. Mechanisms and effects of green tea on cardiovascular health. *Nutrition Reviews.* 2007; 65 (8): 361-375.

[76] Rosenberg IH. Sarcopenia: origins and clinical relevance. *J Nutr.* 1997;127 Suppl:S990–S991.

[77] Cruz-Jentoft AJ, Londi F, Schneider SM, Zumiga C, Arap H, Narie Y, Chein LK, Fielding RA, Martin FC, Michel JP, Sieber C, Stout JR, Studenki AS, Velhas B, Woo J, Zambani M, Ceberholm T. Prevalence of and interventions for sarcopenia in ageing adults: a systematic review. *Report of the International Sarcopenia Initiative (EWGS, OP and IWGS) Ageing and Ageing.* 2014;43:748-759.

[78] International Association of Gerontology and Geriatrics (IAGG) 2011.

[79] Janssen I, Baumgartner RN, Ross R, Rosenberg IH, Roubenoff R. Skeletal Muscle Cutpoints Associated with Elevated Physical Disability Risk in Older Men and Women. *Am J Epidemiol.* 2004 Feb 15; 159(4):413-21.

[80] Chen LK, Liu LK, Woo J, Assotachai P, Auyeung TW, Bahyah KS, Chou MY, Lee Y, Liang C, Limpawattana P, Lin CS, Peng LN, Satake S, Arai H. Consensus report of the Asian Working group for sarcopenia. *Journal of the American Medical Director Association.* 2014; 15(2): 95-101.

[81] Smith AB, Deal Am, Yu H, Boyd B, Matthews J, Wallen EM, Pruthi RS, Woods ME, Muss H, Nielsen ME. Sarcopenia as a predictor of complications and survival Following Radical cystectomy. *The Journal of Urology.* 2014;191(6): 1714-1720.

[82] NIH Consensus Development Panel on Osteoporosis Prevention D, and Therapy. Osteoporosis prevention, diagnosis, and therapy. *JAMA*. 2001;285(6):785–795.

[83] Unnanuntana A, Rebolledo BJ, Khair MM, DiCarlo EF, Lane JM. Diseases affecting bone quality: beyond osteoporosis. *Clin Orthop Relat Res*. 2011;469(8):2194–2206.

[84] Siris ES, Chen YT, Abbott TA, et al. Bone mineral density thresholds for pharmacological intervention to prevent fractures. *Arch Intern Med.* 2004;164(10):1108–1112.

[85] WHO. *Bone and Joint decade.* Available at: www.boneandjoint decade.org, 2008.

[86] Johansson J, Nordström A, Nordström P. Objectively measured physical activity is associated with parameters of bone in 70-year-old men and women. *Bone* 2015;81:72-9.

[87] Sarkar M, Bhardwaj R, Madabhavi I, Khatana J. Osteoporosis in chronic obstructive pulmonary disease. *Clin Med Insights Circ Respir Pulm Med.* 2015;9:5–21.

[88] Okazaki R, Watanabe R, Inoue D. Osteoporosis Associated with Chronic Obstructive Pulmonary Disease. *J. Bone Metab.* 2016;23(3):111-120.

[89] Inoue D, Watanabe R, Okazaki R. COPD and osteoporosis: links, risks, and treatment challenges. *Int J Choron Obstruct. Pulmon Dis.* 2016; 11637-648.

[90] Watanabe R, Tanaka T, Aita K, et al. Osteoporosis is highly prevalent in Japanese males with chronic obstructive pulmonary disease and is associated with deteriorated pulmonary function. *J Bone Miner Metab.* 2015;33(4):392–400.

[91] Decramer M, Janssens W, Miravitlles M. Chronic obstructive pulmonary disease. *Lancet* 2012;379:1341-51.

[92] Lopes MA, Bottino CMC, Hototian SR. Epidemiology of dementias: critical analysis of current evidence. In: Bottino CM, Laks J, Blay SL. *Dementia and cognitive disorders in the elderly*. Rio de Janeiro: Guanabara Koogan; 2006. p. 23-30.

[93] Caixeta L, Nitrini R. Clinical subtypes of frontotemporal dementia. *Arq. Neuropsiquiatr.* 2001;59(3-A): 577-581.

[94] Barker Al, Bird ML, Talevski J. Effect of Pilates Exercise for improving Balance in Older Adults: a systematic review with Meta-analysis. *Archives of Physical Medicine and Rehabilitation.* 2015; 96:715-723.

[95] Bittar RSM, Bottino MA, Simocell L, Venosa AR. Labyrinth disease secondary to disorders of sugar metabolism: reality or fantasy? *Rev. Bras. Otorrinolaringol.* 2004;70(6) 800-805.

[96] Bullo V, Bergamin M, Gobbo S, Sieverdes JC, Zaccaria M, Neunhaeuserer D, Ermolão A. The effect of Pilates exercises training on physical fitness and wellbeing in the elderly: A systematic review for future exercise prescription. *Preventive Medicine.* 2015; 75: 1-11.

[97] Irez GB, Ozdemir A, Evin R, Irez SG, Korkusuz F. Integratıng Pilates exercise into an exercise program for 65+ year-old women to reduce falls. *Journal of Sports Science and Medicine.* 2011; 10: 105-111.

[98] Josephs S, Pratt ML, Meadows EC, Thurmand S, Wagner A. The effectiveness of Pilates on balance and falls in community dwelling older adults. *Journal of Bodywork & Mov. Therap.* 2016; 20:815-823.

[99] Eyigor, S., Karapolat, H., Yesil, H., Uslu, R., & Durmaz, B. (2010). Effects of Pilates exercises on functional capacity, flexibility, fatigue, depression and quality of life in female breast cancer patients: A randomized controlled study. *European Journal of Physical and Rehabilitation Medicine,* 46, 481–487.

[100] Ruddy KJ, Stan DL, Bhagna A, Jurisson M, Cheville AL. Alternative Exercise Traditions in cancer rehabilitation. *Phy Med. Rehabil clin N Am.* 2017; 28:181-192.

[101] Sener HO, Malkoç M, Ergin G, Karadibak D, Yavuzsen T. Effects of clinical Pilates Exercises on Patients Developing lymphedema after Breast cancer Treatment: A randomized clinical trial. *J. Breast Health.* 2017; 13:16-22.

[102] *Pilates styles.* August(4), 2007.

[103] Aladro-Gonzalo AR, Araya-Vargas GA, Machado-Díaz M, Salazar-Rojas W. Pilates based exercise for persistent, non-specific low back pain and associated functional disability: A meta-analysis with meta-regression. *Journal of Bodywork & Mov Therap.* 2013; 17:125-136.

[104] da Luz MA, Costa LO, Fuhro FF, et al. Effectiveness of mat Pilates or equipment-based Pilates in patients with chronic non-specific low back pain: a protocol of a randomised controlled trial. *BMC Musculoskelet Disord* 2013;14:16.

[105] Hayflick, LH. *How and why we grow older.* Rio de Janeiro: Campus, 1996. 400p).

[106] Da Luz MA, Costa LOP, Fuhro FF, Manzani ACT, Oliveira NTB, Cabral CMN. Effectiveness of Mat Pilates or Equipment-Based Pilates Exercise in Patients with Chronic Nonspecific low Back Pain: A randomized controlled trial. *Physical Therapy.* 2014; 94: 623-631.

[107] Cruz-Dias D, Martinez-Amat A, Osuna-Pérez MC, Torrecruz MJ, Hita-Conheras F. Short and long-term effects of a six-week clinical Pilates program in addition to physical therapy on postmenopausal women with chronic low back pain: a randomized controlled trial. *Disability and Rehabilitation.* 2015. http://dx.doi.org/10.3109/0963 8288.2015.1090485.

[108] Royer L, Waldmann K. *Pilates for People with Parkinson 's disease.* Balanced Body Sunner. 2007.

[109] Doidge, N. *The brain's way of healing: remarkable discoveries and recoveries from the frontiers of neuroplasticity.* 2015.

[110] Compston A, Coles A. Multiple Sclerosis. *Lancet.* 2008; 372(9648): 1502-17.

[111] Mc Alpines. *Multiple Sclerosis.* Churchill Livingstone - Elsevier. 2006.

[112] Scalfari A, Neuhaus A, Degenhardt A, Rice GP, Muraro PA, Daumer M, Ebers GC. The natural history of multiple sclerosis a geographically based study 10: Relapses and long-term disability. *Brain.* 2010; 133:1914-1929.

[113] Kuçük F, Kara B, Poyraz EÇ, Idiman E. Improvements in cognition, quality of life, and physical performance with clinical Pilates in

multiple sclerosis: A randomized controlled trial. *Journal of Physical Therapy Science.* 2016;b28:761-788.

[114] Tomkuk MS, Zahid Vz M, Kara B, Idiman E. *Effects of Pilates exercises on sensory interaction, postural control and fatigue in patients with multiple sclerosis and related disorders.* 2016; 7:70-73.

[115] Vanderlinden ML, Bulley C, Geneen LJ, Hooper JE, Cowan P, Mercer TH. Pilates for people with multiple sclerosis who use a wheelchair: Feasibility, efficacy and participant experiences. *Disabil. Rehabil.* 2014; 34(11): 932-939.

[116] Lourenti R. Measurement of quality of life. *Rev. Assoc. Med. Bras.* 2003. http://dx.doi.org/10.1590/50104-42302003000400021.

[117] The WHOQOL Group: The World Health Organization Quality of Life Assessment (WHOQOL): Position paper from the Health Organization. *Soc. Sci. Med,* 1995,41(10):1403-1409.

[118] Caldwell K. Pilates, Mindfulness and Somatic Education. *J. Dance Somat Pract.* 2013; 5(2):141-153.

[119] Kuçük F, Livanelioglu A. Impact of the clinical Pilates exercises and verbal education on exercise beliefs and psychosocial factor in healthy women. *J. Phys. Ther. Sci.* 2015; 27:3437-3443.

[120] Küçükçakir N, Alton L, Karkmoz N. Effects of Pilates exercises on pain, functional status and quality of life in women with postmenopausal osteoporosis. *Journal of Bodywork & Mov. Therap.* 2013; 17:1204-1211.

[121] Natour J, Cazotti LA, Ribeiro LH, Baptista AS, Jones A. Pilates improves pain, function and quality of life in patients with chronic low back pain: a randomized controlled trial. *Clinical Rehabilitation.* 2015; 29(1):59-68.

[122] Campos RR, Dias JM, Pereira LM, Obara RA, Iversen MD, Cardoso JR. Effect of Pilates method on physical conditioning of health subjects: A systematic review and meta-analysis. *The Journal of Sports Medicine and Physical Fitness.* 2016; 56(7-8):864-873.

[123] Rohn SY. The effect of 12-week Pilates exercises on wellness in the elderly. *Journal of Exercise Rehabilitation.* 2016; 12(2): 119-123.

About the Author

Silvana Junges is a Pilates method teacher at the Pilates Silvana Junges Studio in the city of Porto Alegre, RS, Brazil. She has a degree in Physical Education from the Faculty of Health Sciences of Porto Alegre Institute of the Methodist Church. She received her Master's in Medicine and Health Sciences and a PhD in Biomedical Gerontology from the Pontifical Catholic University of Rio Grande do Sul, RS, Brazil. She currently researches and writes about the benefits of the Pilates method in the elderly. She is a reviewer of the journal *Scientia Medica*. She is now volunteering at a project in Nepal with elderly people in need.

INDEX

A

B

C

D